THE
SUCCESS-
ENERGY
EQUATION

HOW TO REGAIN FOCUS, RECHARGE YOUR LIFE + REALLY GET SH!T DONE

THE SUCCESS-ENERGY EQUATION

MICHELLE CEDERBERG

● ● **PAGE TWO** BOOKS

Cataloguing in publication information is available from Library and Archives Canada.
ISBN 978-1-77458-020-2 (paperback)
ISBN 978-1-77458-021-9 (ebook)

Produced by Page Two
www.pagetwo.com

Edited by Kendra Ward
Copyedited by Melissa Edwards
Cover design by Jennifer Lum
Interior design by Fiona Lee

www.michellecederberg.com

To my octogenarian mother, Britta, whose healthy, happy approach to life has always been fueled by boundless common sense, and more science smarts than she knows.

You taught me well, Mom!

CONTENTS

Introduction: How We Work Isn't Working 1

PART I **REGAIN FOCUS, RECHARGE YOUR LIFE**

1 21st-and-a-Quarter-Century Stress 13

2 A Simpler Equation 33

3 Stuck on Autopilot 49

4 From Autopilot to Awareness 67

PART II **READY, SET, GOALS**

5 Good Goals, Great Gains 89

6 Manage Your Motivation Matrix 109

7 Build Belief in Yourself and Your Goals 123

PART III **REALLY GET SH!T DONE**

8 Unleash Discipline 153

9 Energy as a Magic Multiplier of Success 171

10 The Success-Energy Connection 195

Acknowledgments 205

Notes 209

INTRODUCTION

HOW WE WORK ISN'T WORKING

THE WORLD WE live in is demanding more from us than ever before. Do you feel it?

We're tasked with the daily responsibilities of work and life—job, family, friends, home obligations, finances, health—just like our parents were, and their parents before that. Today, though, the added overwhelm of technology is linked to everything we do. We race through the day with our eyeballs glued to a high-powered computer while our fingers swipe and tap, swipe and tap. We call it a smartphone, but really, why would we make an actual phone call when we can tweet, text, email, and use Messenger, Snapchat, TikTok, WhatsApp, or Instagram no matter the time of day or what we happen to be doing at the moment?

And these days our news feeds are besieged with the heaviness of the twenty-four-hour news cycle: politics, war, the economy, poverty, climate change, racism, terrorism, and global health crises. World news has never been so accessible and pervasive, and some days the weight of that information overload can be too much.

We've got devices and apps to track our health, wealth, productivity, or lack of it. We'll hear a reminder buzz if we go off track. We've got so many distractions available at the swipe of a finger that days can go by with little attention paid to the real world and the people in it. So, we develop a relationship with our voice-controlled personal assistant, who listens in on our lives and automates everything from checking the weather to calling the kids to dinner.

"Alexa, help me make sense of it all!"

We're overburdened—mentally, physically, emotionally, and cognitively—with all we're forced to sort through on any given day. One could argue that overwhelm has always been a part of life. The world has forever tossed challenges our way, and we've done our best to juggle them. The addition of technological distractions has only added to the chaos. It has hijacked our precious bandwidth and stolen any bit of restorative downtime we thought we had. And it's changed how we work.

Which is why I wrote *The Success-Energy Equation*—to share ideas and information that will help you navigate today's new brand of overwhelm and clarify what you want more of in your work and life. You'll also learn how to go after it. And my methods may surprise you.

In a world that is overpoweringly complex and automated, where we're increasingly busy and overloaded by life, this book encourages a shift toward simplicity. Now, more than ever, the path to success requires a return to the basics so we can rise above the noise. No, I don't want to you to throw away your smartphone and live off the grid, but I do want you to get smart about the ways in which technology and the pace of life affect how you work. I want you to understand how your body functions under what I call 21st-and-a-quarter-century stress, and how to restore yourself in ways that combat that pressure. I share methods that will help you get clear, confident, and disciplined for the parts of work and life that truly matter to you.

The principles I teach in this book rely on two truths: what science says about health and human performance, and the deep-down common sense you already possess about what it takes to find success. This combination is more powerful than you know, and it will help you work better. At everything.

We get only one chance to do *this* life, to be fully present in it, to make the most of it. And since none of us will really know for sure whether reincarnation exists until we've left this "mortal coil," let's go with that notion. One life. One chance to do the freakin' work ... or, more precisely, to do the *right* work on the *right* things *right now* to create a life that you love. Are you kicking butt and taking numbers? I hope so, because life should be full of success, fun, and fulfillment. If *your* life is, keep reading so you can add to that success.

And if life feels unfulfilling or you're a bit fried, it happens. Sometimes life does feel like work. Because we, as busy, driven people—in our striving for achievement—unwittingly do one thing that limits our capacity for success, even though we're doing it to stay on top of things. In our quest to get everything done, we each have a day-in-day-out routine that we initiate without thinking. As a defense against the endless demands of our lives, we rush through the day on autopilot—making unconscious, automatic decisions that don't necessarily align with how we want to work and live.

Get up, eat, work, eat, sleep, repeat. Get up, eat, get the kids going, work, eat, work out, sleep, repeat. Get up, eat, walk the dog, work, work, work, eat, sleep, repeat. The variables change from person to person, and likely there are a lot more of them than those I've listed, but you get the drift. Get up, *do life*, sleep, repeat ... day after day after day. Often until you're tired, burned out, overwhelmed, and stressed.

You're busy, so you must be making progress, right? But in the frenzy of the day, it's probably not your best work, it might not be the right work, and that pace comes at cost. Autopilot will eventually impact your ability to have fun, and to effectively and efficiently get work done. Perhaps it already has.

In an ideal, *less chaotic* world you might shift into autopilot for a "short flight" now and then, during a particularly busy day or week, but if autopilot is your normal, watch out. Humans on autopilot don't work as well as airplanes on autopilot. This control mechanism will slow your progress forward and stop you from going in the direction you're truly meant to travel. And if you stay in that flight mode too long, you'll go off course. You'll lose sight of what is truly important. You'll get lost. Autopilot is purely a survival tactic, and it's *not* how we work best.

If you feel like you're going through the motions some days (or many), if life feels too routine or a bit mundane, if distractions are draining your energy, if you're constantly rushing out the door, rushing to get it all done, wondering when you'll find a bit of calm, or feeling the chaos of life, then it might be time to get present to the mess. That 21st-and-a-quarter-century stress may be impacting your success.

So much of success comes down to human performance and your capacity to operate at a high level—mentally, physically, and emotionally—no matter what comes at you. Today's brand of high-level stress, endless distractions, and lack of time management means we go through life ignoring what we need for ourselves in those areas. As an antidote to 21st-and-a-quarter-century stress, you need to slow down and start listening to your body again. It knows what you need.

The Success-Energy Equation will help you do just that. It explores 21st-and-a-quarter-century stress and what you must do to push past it toward a life of greater clarity, confidence, and success. It's about how your physical body and the brilliant mind in it work to help you work better . . . if you just pay attention to what it's telling you.

Presence and Clarity

The Success-Energy Equation asks you to get present to your life as it is right now and clarify what you want. When life is busy and you're just doing your best to keep it all together, it's easy to lose direction with your goals because you don't have the time or energy to pursue them. Heck, there's no time to think about them, let alone pursue them.

What's working? What's not? What inspires you to jump into each day? What goals do you have for your work and life? This book will remind you of the importance of goals as you strive for better, and it will inspire you to set worthwhile goals that will help you work smarter, and with more focus and fulfillment. Purpose is a powerful driver of success, and when you're clear about yours, great things are possible.

The Success-Energy Equation also addresses how attitude, self-confidence, and self-efficacy contribute to success. How you choose to work and what you choose to work at are guided by your mindset and belief systems, and when you can own the fact that you deserve success and are capable of doing the work, that empowerment will greatly influence how much you achieve.

The Success-Energy Equation explores *how* we work at anything we work at—our discipline for doing the work. It looks at the good, the bad, and the ugly of the daily habits we default to, and how they impact our ability to do everything better. What do you do well, where do you fall short, and how can you strengthen your discipline? Productivity can increase in magical ways with even small shifts in how you work.

Perhaps most importantly, *The Success-Energy Equation* reminds you that a focus on health and energy management will not only sustain your efforts in all you do but also drive you toward higher levels of success. Energy is the *magic multiplier* for goals, mindset, and discipline, and it's your not-so-secret weapon against 21st-and-a-quarter-century stress.

At the end of every chapter, you'll find a short segment called "Engage Your #SuccessEnergy" where I ask you to answer a few questions or do an assessment. You'll have just read the chapter, and you'll want the information to stick, right? This will happen more effectively if you do a bit of homework around it before you move on to the next chapter. You'll have the opportunity to think about how the information applies specifically to you, and how you'll improve your energy. For maximum impact, don't skip these sections. In fact, research supports notetaking to enhance learning and retention,[1] so it might be a good idea to keep a journal or notebook handy as you read through the book to answer the questions and track your progress in one place.

Peppered throughout the book you'll find a number of special sections that share interesting ideas and facts. Your physical body and the brilliant mind in it are truly amazing pieces of human machinery that will help you do everything better, if you know what to look for, and if you pay attention to what they need throughout the day. These segments impart some of the wonderful ways your body works to help you work better, backed by new scientific research and by what science already knows to be true about human performance. Did I say fascinating? Yup, fascinating!

The Payoff

When tapped into properly, health and energy management ensures higher levels of focus, confidence, happiness, and success—not to mention longevity and health. Yet when life gets busy, we ignore our physiological needs and inadvertently push self-care to the side, perhaps justifying that the work in front of us is more important than rest or movement or leisure time. That's not how your body works. Not at its best, anyway.

Energy management needs to be a part of your non-negotiable success strategy. How you do everything works so much better when you remember that your body is the machine that drives the mission. With that in mind, this book shares all of the awesome productivity-boosting, idea-generating, confidence-enhancing, clarity-creating benefits that health and energy bring to your work and to everything that is important to you.

In this moment, think about what you truly want for yourself in your work and your life, then trust that *The Success-Energy Equation* will support you, if you're willing to do the work.

This book will show you how to get the clarity, courage, work ethic, and energy it takes to create the life you want. Whether you're a driven decision-maker, an empire-building entrepreneur, or a pulled-in-every-direction parent—heck, if you're retired, tired, or uninspired—you were put on this planet to make your mark, well and enthusiastically. I want to help you do just that.

Read on with an openness to what's possible for you, if you do the work. Every ounce of effort will be worth it. Carpe Freakin' Diem!

PART I

REGAIN FOCUS, RECHARGE YOUR LIFE

1

21ST-AND-A-QUARTER-CENTURY STRESS

---

66 Be ambitious. Get shit done.
Keep your priorities straight, your mind
right, and your head up. 99

AUTHOR UNKNOWN

AS I WAS formulating ideas for this book, I spent a lot of time thinking about success and the ways we hold ourselves back from doing the things we're truly capable of. Even when we know what we want, we don't always do what it takes to get it. We set common sense aside and we procrastinate, we prioritize poorly or amuse ourselves with distractions, we let other people influence our actions, we doubt ourselves. And yet, despite this truth, we all strive, every day, to work hard and live the best possible life. Perhaps we underestimate how much stress may be affecting our success.

Life is busy. It's an overused statement, but only because it's so freakin' true. Crazy and conflicting family schedules, long work hours, and heavy workloads are only part of the problem. We're living in the twenty-first century, the most technologically advanced time in history. And although computers and devices have improved our lives in many ways and most of us can't imagine living without our smartphones, that connectedness influences our stress levels, our relationships, and our overall health and well-being. (Excuse me a second while I check my phone.)

I call it 21st-and-a-quarter-century stress, which is a pervasive, unrelenting, tech-driven, FOMO-fed stress that has us on the go—physically, mentally, emotionally, even cognitively—all day long. For many of us, the madness begins in the grogginess of early morning as we fumble for the light of the smartphone and scroll through the cyber-world as our first entry point into the day.

We're living in an age of hyper-connectedness, checking work emails at all hours, texting when we should be talking, surfing mindlessly when we have a spare moment, scrolling other people's lives instead of living our own, or fanatically nurturing our online lives for an audience of pseudo friends; we're letting our self-esteem drop with every comparison to their perfect, edited, selfie-catalogued lives.

Maybe you eat breakfast, maybe you don't. About 40 percent of North Americans skip breakfast. Most say it's because they aren't hungry (42 percent), or they simply don't have time (38 percent). In the short term, that morning fast impacts energy and focus. In the long term it could have a negative effect on weight and other undesirable health consequences. Of the 60 percent who do eat breakfast, 21 percent eat grab-and-go meals because of time constraints.

You probably have time to eat in your car, though. Traffic density in most major cities means we're spending more and more time commuting, stuck in traffic, whiling away hours in our cars or on trains or subways. The average one-way commute in North America is between twenty-six and twenty-nine minutes. That's almost an hour per day of unproductive, mind-numbing time lost to coming and going. Sixty minutes a day, five days a week, forty-eight weeks per year adds up to 240 hours, or ten full days of each year spent commuting to and from work. Think of all the things you could do with that time.

I asked that very question of clients, friends, and colleagues in an informal social media poll: *If you had an extra hour each day, how would you use it?* The top three responses were, in order of popularity, (1) I'd sleep more, (2) I'd get more exercise, and (3) I'd do fun things more often. All of which are infinitely better than sucking exhaust fumes in stop-and-go traffic, and all speak to the ongoing deficiencies in our routines.

When you take vacation days (if you do), you likely find it increasingly difficult to truly disconnect and unwind. According to a U.K. survey of one thousand people, 52 percent of employees check work emails during vacation.[1] A Randstad survey reported that 42 percent of employees feel "obligated" to do so, and 26 percent feel guilty using all their vacation time.[2] Most of us are connected to work, social media, and all things digital even when we're meant to relax and rejuvenate.

At work you navigate deadlines, obnoxious co-workers, nerve-wracking presentations, unnecessary meetings, and the constant buzz of new email alerts and text messages. And you may even wish you weren't there. According to the 2017 Gallup worker satisfaction survey, 85 percent of employees are either not engaged or are actively disengaged at work.[3] We're giving our time to the grind, but not our best effort and ideas. No time for breaks, or, if we take them, we numb out in the digital space (like, like, winky emoji, heart, wow) and eat lunch at our desks. Throughout the day we're afflicted with information overload from all the social media notifications, or with FOMO if we don't check in and respond. We're weighed down by the heaviness of world news, politics, climate change, and the economy.

With all this going on, it probably occurs to you more than once a day that it's a mad, mad, mad, world.

Maybe you work out, maybe you don't. No time or energy, but either way all that sitting has a negative impact on your health, not to mention brain output. You'd like to work out more. Who wouldn't? But first thing in the morning doesn't appeal to your sleep-deprived body, there's never enough time at lunch (besides, you have too much work to catch up on), and after work you've got last-minute errands, or have to pick up the kids, or get dinner on the table. You walk a bit, though, and do a spin class once a week, and every now and then you channel your inner weekend warrior with a hike or a ski day, which you feel for days after.

Once you get home at the end of your busy, stressful, distraction-filled day, it dawns on you that you haven't had two minutes to yourself, and you're not entirely certain what that even feels like anymore. You've still got to feed the family, care for your kids, pets, partner, all the above or none of the above, and if it's the latter you need to figure out why you're single, and how you can change it without having to resort to swipe left or right dating options.

As you get ready for bed—later than you hoped because you had to make lunches, do laundry, check emails (or your online dating options)—you take stock of your non-stop, go-big-or-go-home, get-shit-done day. You had hoped today would be different. You planned to get more done. But just like yesterday, and the day before that, you didn't accomplish half of what you thought you would at work, and you haven't had time to have much of a life.

Welcome to 21st-and-a-quarter-century stress. It could be messing with your success.

Each day, as you strive for better, not only must you get through the curves and roadblocks of everyday life, you must also navigate the unknown: the barriers that are out of your control, the barricades that others toss in your way, even the mental and emotional blocks, real or perceived, that you create for yourself. This, while juggling distractions from the digital space and energy-drains from an increasingly dysfunctional and demanding world. Our bodies are tired, our brains are full, and our capacity is being tested.

Common Sense Is Stronger with Science

Deep down we all possess good sense about what will help us be healthy, happy, and successful. We understand right from wrong, healthy from unhealthy, productive versus wasteful, useful versus useless, yet knowing better doesn't mean we always do better.

Common sense—having good sense and sound judgment in practical matters—as the old saying goes, isn't very common.[4] That's too bad, because if we tapped into it more often, it could help drive our success. It's *because* common sense isn't always common practice that we need reminders for *why* we should do the work or set aside distractions or make better choices. Enter science.

Common sense strengthens when our sound judgment is supported by painstaking scientific study of why it matters, and that it works. And since you may not get as excited about digging through all the research as I do, I've done a lot of it for you. You'll find the results throughout this book, and in special sections like this one. I'm hoping that when you read the science behind the success strategies in this book, it will teach you something new, or reinforce what you already know to be true, and perhaps remind you *why* it matters. It should also provide a bit of insurance: that if you choose to invest the time and energy to do the work, you'll get the results. This is how you can use science and common sense to do everything better.

Acute, Chronic, or Pervasive?

Typically, we categorize stress in two ways: acute or chronic. Acute stress is single-bout, short-term stress, like a tough day at work, a moment of conflict with your boss, a traffic jam, or an argument with your teenager. While the stressor is present, you'll experience typical stress responses like increased blood pressure and heart rate, increased gut and muscle tension, and a higher breathing rate—and you probably won't feel happy. Then the tough workday will end, or the conflict will, or you'll get out of traffic, or your teenager will stomp off to their room, you'll take a deep breath, and your body will begin to recover from the stress. Eventually you'll start to breathe more normally, your heart rate will slow down, and you'll feel less tense. Acute stress is stress with adequate recovery and it's how we're meant to work.

Chronic stress is long-term stress, or stress without adequate recovery. You're probably pretty good at navigating the odd tough day at the office, or the occasional run-in with your boss, but if every day is a tough day, or the drive home is always traffic-clogged, or your home life is fraught with family arguments (or all of the above), recovery from stress will be difficult. If the body doesn't get a chance to recover from stressful situations, it creates a new normal. The common markers of stress—increases in heart rate, blood pressure, breathing, gut and muscle tension, even cortisol levels—stay elevated, so your body must work harder to help you function normally. If chronic stress is prolonged it can lead to stress-related health problems like high blood pressure, diabetes, heart disease, ulcers, chronic pain, or depression.

So, how is 21st-and-a-quarter-century stress different from chronic stress? In many ways, it isn't. It *is* long-term stress without adequate recovery. It *is* ever-present, in myriad forms, just like chronic stress, but I propose that it is more pervasive, because we are connected 24/7 to the digital space—to news (fake or otherwise), social media, apps, games, streaming programs, videos, shopping, pop-up ads, emails, text messages, and any number of alerts. Plus, we can access work-related information at all hours of the day, so our workday has no boundaries.

While technology has enhanced many aspects of our work and life, the bandwidth overload it creates is affecting us—body, mind, and spirit—like never before. Every day we're tasked with navigating all that is happening in our physical world, with the added burden of processing the digital noise inundating us from the online space and the little supercomputer we call a smartphone.

This daily physical-digital juggling act means your body and mind both lack recovery time. The pervasive stress that happens *to us* as digital information gets pushed into our devices—and that we perpetuate through our dependence on these devices—creates 21st-and-a-quarter-century stress. A modern-day offshoot of chronic stress, it is a relatively new phenomenon.

When the first compact mobile phones hit the market in the early nineties, all you could really do with them was make phone calls or tap out a rudimentary text, but it meant you didn't have to find a pay phone or landline to make a call, and you didn't have to go home to listen to the messages on your answering machine. Since life was busy back then too, we embraced the convenience. The mobile phone became the gateway device for what was to follow, because if you had one, every time you upgraded to a new one there were more bells and whistles.

The smartphone was first introduced in the nineties, but it didn't truly come of age until 2007, when Steve Jobs announced the impending availability of the iPhone at the Macworld conference. The device was released for sale in June of that year, and people lined up outside stores to buy one. Apple sold 270,000 iPhones the first weekend it was available, and by Labor Day sales had reached one million. I think you'd agree that, from that point on, consumers never looked back.

The number of smartphone users worldwide is projected to total 3.8 billion by 2021, marking an 11.8 percent increase from 2019.[5] The number increased by one billion between 2016 and 2020 alone. With the global population at 7.7 billion, that means 45.4 percent of the people on this planet have a smartphone. In 2020 more than five billion people in the world own a mobile device of some sort. That number is projected to increase to 7.33 billion by 2023.

China, India, and the United States lead the world in smartphone use. In 2020 it is estimated that 83 percent of Americans and 81 percent of Canadians own a smartphone.[6] That translates to about 270 million distracted, zoned out users in the U.S. and 28 million in Canada. We're connected globally and to all things digital, and disconnected with what is happening right around us. It's a lot to process. Literally.

Although devices are a big part of 21st-and-a-quarter-century stress, you're not entirely immune if you're one of those rare individuals without a smartphone tethered to your body. Unless you're living in a completely tech-free world, information overload can happen via your computer, your television, or the information that bombards you during your day: non-stop news cycles, computer pop-ups, social media posts, advertising, emails, and so on. Heck, when you walk through a crowded food court or airport and observe everyone with their noses in their phones, your stress levels may rise from the insanity of it all. The content of world news is more stressful these days too, with climate change, terrorism, war, racial tensions, pandemics, fake news, bad news, and absurd politics.

It's all around us and it's not going away, but it's neither wise nor beneficial to simply habituate to the noise and tune out the physical world around us. So, what now?

First, Get Clear

If you can identify with the busyness that is 21st-and-a-quarter-century stress, and if you're feeling a bit lost because of it, the road to lower levels of stress and higher levels of success may be difficult to find at first. Maybe you're too tired or too busy doing life to contemplate possibilities. Or it hasn't occurred to you that change is possible. Or you know that it is, but you can't imagine where you'll find the time or energy to do what it takes. That's the influence of 21st-and-a-quarter-century stress on your life. It draws down your mental, physical, emotional, and cognitive bandwidth until you lose sight of what is truly important to you. And since the goal of this book is to help you mitigate this kind of stress so that you can get to success, a great first step is to clarify what success looks like for you. This process starts with a question:

What do you want?

Most professional coaches use this simple but powerful question to help clients get clear. I call it the "big little question" because, while it's simple, it requires you to dig in and think deeply about where you are now and where you want to go with your life. What do *you* want for yourself, separate from everyone else, including your family, your boss, your parents, your friends? What do you want more of, what have you been missing, what can you do without? This fully loaded question is not always easy to answer quickly, but once you do, your "path to next" will light up and you'll feel excited for what's possible.

The problem is, with life being so busy, and with screen time filling the extra space, we don't give ourselves the opportunity to ponder possibilities, or we're so distracted we fail to pay attention to what head and heart are yearning for. So, start thinking about the answer to that question right now.

What do you want?

If you think about it, what most of us want out of life is some version of the following: *to be healthy, happy, and financially stress-free.* You might say this is an oversimplified definition of success, but if you think about what matters to you, your goals, and the ways you'd like to improve your work and life, your responses likely lean toward some version of healthier, happier, and financially stress-free.

This simple definition doesn't make the achievement of success any easier, though, as there are so many different yet acceptable interpretations of healthier, happier, and financially stress-free. Your health may fall somewhere on the spectrum from super-fit, plant-based, booze-free, sugar-free, stress-free to "I'm unhealthy and I need to do something about it." Most of us fall somewhere between the extremes. Do you feel good about your health practices? At the minimum, if you take care of exercise, sleep, stress, and nutrition in a way that ensures longevity and gives you the energy and focus to conquer all you must do and want to do, you've got success with your health.

Happiness is so wide open to interpretation that examples would fill an entire book. Do you know what makes you happiest and do you have that in your life? If you get up most days and feel content with the people, circumstances, and opportunities that surround you, you've got success with your happiness.

Financially stress-free is about being able to pay your bills and ensure your basic needs are met. This is perhaps the most challenging success indicator in North America, where as many as 53 percent of Canadians live paycheck to paycheck[7] and more than 74 percent of employees in America would experience financial difficulty if their paychecks were delayed for a week.[8] And we're not saving as much as we should.

In an ideal world, we'd all have high-paying jobs, with ample savings in the bank, money to cover the cost of living, and extra to enjoy life a little bit. In reality, many people struggle financially in one or all of these areas, and financially stress-free may simply mean learning to live within your means and improving your financial situation as much as possible. Some people want it all and won't stop until they get it, while others can happily live on very little—and at the very least, if basic needs are met, that can be enough. What are you striving toward?

Although each of us has a very different idea of what success should look like, most of us crave health, happiness, and financial stability, all at the same time.

You can't *really* call it success if one of these areas is suffering. You may have built a great career and bank balance to the detriment of your health and family life, or you could have a great relationship and good health but can't make ends meet. And where does that leave you? Or you have a "dream job" but you're ridiculously unhappy in it. Or everything in your life may be amazing, and then your health or the health of a loved one shakes the foundation. Or you have a rewarding career, and enough money, but you're unlucky in love and unhappy because of it. Or you lose a chunk of your retirement savings, or you lose your job. You get the drift. Life works best when all three work well. If you're clear on that point, great things are possible.

When you think about what happy, healthy, and financially stress-free looks like for you, where are the gaps? Which areas of your life need your attention? Which areas are you most drawn to improving, and, perhaps a better question to ask: What's stopping you?

Next, What's Stopping You?

As an encouraging motivational speaker and professional coach, I genuinely believe that people are capable of so much more than they give themselves credit for. I want people to recognize their strengths and summon the courage to create the life and career they truly want.

This starts with *knowing* what you want, and from there you have to do the work. So, if there is a formula for success, it may be as simple as this:

THE DREAM × HARD WORK = SUCCESS

In theory, this equation is fantastic: Do the freakin' work, get the freakin' results, right? You've identified the dream and you're prepared to do the work. In your mind's eye you can see what success will look like, and it looks great. You envision how you'll feel when you achieve your goals. Amazing! You believe reaching them is possible and you know what you need to do. You're probably doing a bit of it already, and you have the best of intentions to keep at it. You're excited about your future!

But putting all the elements into practice and maintaining momentum, day in and day out, is a lot harder than you thought it would be. Success is hard. That's life.

We can't really blame ourselves for getting caught up in the hope this equation conjures. After all, many people have found success via this formula, haven't they? Plus, success gurus and overzealous motivational types with limitless energy and nothing in the way regularly thrust this idea upon us. *It's yours for the taking. Decide what you want and then reach for the stars. The world is waiting for you. Clap if you're with me!* Surely they're not making this stuff up?

Enter the pragmatic motivational speaker. I'm here to remind you that it's not that simple, because as you drive the road to success life will toss a lot of barriers in front of you, and you need to be prepared for them. External circumstances out of your control—like the economy, weather events, accidents, job loss, other people, and even workload at times—might present challenges. Or external circumstances within your control—like where you live or work, your health and financial habits, the distractions you indulge in, or the quality of your relationships—could present as barriers to your success. And then there are the internal views and thought processes that hold you back—like your limiting beliefs, self-doubt, and lack of self-confidence.

I'm not trying to be a killjoy. The pragmatist in me needs to remind you of the barriers, not so that you give up trying, but so that you can do the work with eyes wide open, shoulders squared, and inner strength reinforced. This truth will increase your chances of success at anything you do.

If the realities of everyday life don't factor into your formula for success, you'll set yourself up for less than what you deserve. Your brain will hijack your efforts: *Why can't I do this? I'm not smart enough, there's not enough time, I don't have the skill, I've got bad genes, I'm too busy, I don't know the right people, I've got no support . . . blah, blah, blah.* Or events outside your control will get in the way. Or other people will.

Even still, you deserve whatever it is you dream for yourself. And, yes, you can get there through hard work, but it's also important to open your eyes to all the factors that contribute to that work. Then, as you navigate your own unique path to success, you'll be better equipped to overcome more of the barriers.

Here's my pragmatist version of the formula for success, and admittedly, a scenario that has played out in my own life more than once. See if you can relate. That equation—"the dream × hard work = success"—looks more like this:

The dream × gaining skill + knowledge × hard work = success. Then divide that by days grinding it out, minus time spent on distractions, but add to that persistence, passion, and focus. Then subtract sleep, which equals no energy (to the power of fast food and not exercising), plus patience (to the power of caffeine and anxiety meds) and multiply all that by days spent in self-doubt. That equals stalling. Then you add in an injection of confidence from watching someone else fall on their face. You add in a little bit of guilt for feeling that way, and that equals a reminder to quit comparing your journey with everyone else's, which equals a renewed belief that you can! Multiply all of that by a few days of great progress. Add in fatigue, divide that by more distractions (to the power of whining, complaining, and overthinking), add in more self-doubt, plus roadblocks from your boss, your business partner, your clients, or yourself. That adds up to a drop in motivation, which reduces you to binge-watching Netflix plus wine straight from the bottle. This equals sleeping it off plus an opportunity to rethink your goals, which equals a recommitment to the dream! Divide that by fear about the current economy/weather/government/fill-in-the-blank. Multiply that by optimism, add in vision, plus long hours, plus setbacks (always setbacks), plus resilience, plus drive, multiplied by a desperate need to pay the bills. Add support from loved ones, plus nagging from the same loved ones (which is actually a negative). Subtract frivolity, subtract downtime, subtract holidays. Subtract time or money, subtract sleeping in, subtract leaving work at work, subtract health, add in even more self-doubt, and subtract energy. Through all of this, your efforts are multiplied by a hope that it's possible and a deep-down belief that you can, and that is the real formula for success to the power of WTF!?

How many of these barriers have you stared down on your road to better? If my bad-math formula for success is good for anything beyond a chuckle, it's a reminder that success is not meant to be easy. As you navigate through life, so many barriers will pop up and attempt to mess with your success. They could be physical, emotional, social, small, large, or absurd. Some will be tossed out by situations beyond your control, some by people who don't align with your agenda or who want something different for or from you. You yourself will throw up many barriers: self-doubt, fatigue, distractions, an over-full schedule. Of all these roadblocks, the ones that take you down will often surprise you.

If you're chasing something worthwhile, the path to success rarely follows a straight line. It's usually scattered with bumps and barriers and full-on mountains that you'll have to walk around or tunnel through or climb over. And even though you want the success that's on the other side, summoning up the energy or courage or time to get past the obstructions is not always easy. The intricacies of life—the things that make it worthwhile and interesting, really—complicate our way forward. On top of it all, today you also have to navigate the noise of 21st-and-a-quarter-century stress.

We want it to be easy, but it's not. That's life.

The chaos doesn't mean you're failing. The chaos is life with all of its highs and lows and in-your-face challenges that add color and flavor to the journey. The game-changer is what you do to manage the chaos. I've said it before: the world is demanding more from us than it ever has, and we need to find a different way to meet those demands.

Engage Your #SuccessEnergy: Barrier I.D.

In writing this book, I was forever coming up against my own good advice. The goal was clear: write a book on how to work better at everything, with more focus and fulfillment, and with the energy to do so at a higher level. From there, I had to strengthen my own belief systems and discipline in bringing that goal to completion. I fought against countless barriers and excuses—*too tired, too much other stuff to do, work travel, distracted by social media or easier projects or my dog or laundry, ineffective scheduling, not making writing a priority, self-doubt that feeds procrastination*—and it wasn't until I identified those barriers that I could work to get over them.

Not surprisingly, I realized that when I manage my energy better, I work better. I do my best work first thing in the morning, which means if I'm writing, I need to get to bed at a decent hour the night before, preferably having consumed little or no alcohol. Then, when I wake up, I have a glass of water, a small breakfast, and a cup of coffee, which I take straight to my desk.

And since I'm easily distracted by what's in front of me, the night before, I clear my desk of clutter and open my writing on my computer so it's ready to go the moment I sit down. I also turn off my phone or leave it in another room, and I certainly do not check email before that first writing session.

Finally, back when I was a devoted doggie-mama, once Lilly-dog had her breakfast and had been outside, I tried to put my own needs ahead of hers for an hour or two, no matter how earnestly she asked for her walkies. As my husband regularly reminded me, "Michelle, she's a dog. She'll be fine if she has to wait."

Even small barriers can trip you up if you're not paying attention, but once you can recognize them, most are surprisingly surmountable. If you allow yourself to be completely honest, what gets in the way of going after what you truly want? Think about that now because you can't change what you don't admit. We'll dig deeper with barriers as you progress through the chapters, and this quick exercise will allow you to bring some of them forward to think about as you read on, so be ruthless in your assessment. Get clear, get honest, and engage your #SuccessEnergy.

What barriers commonly block your path forward?
Which ones do you have control over?
How will you adjust?

2

A SIMPLER EQUATION

" It is a rough road that leads to
the heights of greatness. "

SENECA

THE BUSYNESS, DISORDER, and distraction that are so prevalent with 21st-and-a-quarter-century stress won't go away without a bit of mindfulness. To address the stress and get to success, you must first step back before you move up. You must take a fresh look at your life as it is right now, clear away a bit of the unnecessary life clutter, and decide what is truly important to you.

You can get there with the help of four key variables that, when working well, will propel you upward in everything you do. Everything.

My simpler formula for success, The Success-Energy Equation, looks like this:

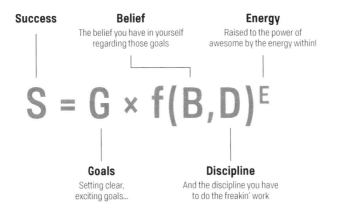

Success

Belief
The belief you have in yourself regarding those goals

Energy
Raised to the power of awesome by the energy within!

$$S = G \times f(B,D)^E$$

Goals
Setting clear, exciting goals...

Discipline
And the discipline you have to do the freakin' work

In this formula S represents success, however you define it for yourself, and it begins with goals (G). We're not talking *set and forget* goals with this formula, we're talking *decide and conquer* goals. Once you've figured out what those goals are, the achievement of them becomes a function (f) of the belief (B) you have in yourself regarding those goals, and the discipline (D) you have within you to do the freakin' work to achieve them.

Of course, there's also that final variable of energy management (E) to address. To put it in math terms, E is the difference-making exponent that will raise those base dreams to the power of awesome. But most people don't include it in their formula for success. Not in the way they should, anyway.

Here's one big reason: You can get by without energy. You can get by without taking care of your health, managing your stress, or tending to your relaxation needs. You can find success even if you eat poorly, don't exercise, smoke, drink too much, sleep poorly, have high stress and no life balance. Many of us do. And since most people have decided they don't have the time or motivation for health anyway, that theory has been proved. Many achieve high levels of success simply by deciding what they want, believing that they can, and doing the work to get it. Health be damned. That equation looks like: $S = G \times f(B,D)$. Period.

So why bother? Why bother doing everything necessary to take care of health and manage energy if you can find success without it? I've got three significant reasons:

Quality of life

You may get to high levels of success without E, but at what cost? What good is success, fame, and fortune if you've let your health slide, or there's no life outside work, or you've neglected important relationships in the process? You're successful, but you're sad, lonely, out of shape, or all the above.

Quality of success

If you're currently knocking it out of the park with career and life success and you're *not* taking care of E, imagine how that success could be multiplied if you did?

Probability of success

Despite being smart, driven, and capable, many people aren't getting to success through belief and hard work alone. Or, perhaps more accurately, to get to success the variables of belief and discipline need a bit of strengthening, which becomes more probable when you embrace the power of E.

AND IF these three reasons aren't enough, when you prioritize E you also increase your physical, mental, emotional, *and* cognitive capacity to deal with the ever-invasive, distracting, pervasive 21st-and-a-quarter-century stress. The key is in E.

Kickstarting Energy

Wherever you are on your success journey, health and energy management (E) will make it better. Yes, the physical body is a stubborn and resilient physiological machine. It will endure through a lot of mistreatment and still drive you toward success, but it has its limits. So why not give it some love before you reach them?

When you include health and energy management as part of your own Success-Energy Equation, you strengthen not only personal health and vitality, but also so many of the drivers of success that have been weakened by 21st-and-a-quarter-century stress. The byproducts of great energy will flow through everything you do and help you be happier, healthier, and more successful. It's such a game-changer that I'm surprised more people don't tap into it.

I recently ran into a colleague whom I hadn't seen in years. I recognized him right away as he walked into the conference hall, but something about him had changed. He'd clearly lost weight, but it was more than that. The Travis I knew from years ago was a funny, gregarious guy who drew people in with his silliness and big smile. At 6-foot-5 and 270 pounds, he had an imposing physique to match his boisterous energy, and he was all about making people smile—an ally, not an intimidator. This new Travis carried himself differently. His goofiness had been replaced with self-assuredness. He seemed to own his space and attracted people to him with his calm energy and confidence. He was happier, healthier, thirty-five pounds lighter, and very much a new man. I was taken by his transformation, so I asked him about it.

Travis's wry answer to my question was, "I got divorced!" Then he explained that his marriage had been shaky for many years and, as a self-confessed people-pleaser in an off-balance relationship, he'd given up a lot of his personal and professional goals to accommodate his wife. Over the years, he'd lost his identity, sense of purpose, and personal power. He was in a miserable marriage and his kids were unhappy because of it. His work didn't inspire him. He'd let his health go, and something needed to change. His answer to the big little question—what do you want?—led him to himself.

His journey back to himself began before his divorce, when he signed up for a twenty-one-day fitness challenge to kick-start his physical health. When you're feeling stuck in life, fitness is often a great place to start because the physical exertion requires energy, but not *emotional* energy. You can just take out your frustrations on the bike or the punching bag or the weights. And it's empowering. He also started seeing a counselor to nurture his spiritual health, which led him to listen more carefully to his own head and heart about what he truly needed for himself.

Travis decided he needed to invest more meaningfully in his business, his health, his relationships, and his kids. He downsized his home, which increased his bank balance, and then spent a lot of time getting rid of the excess weight of "things" in his life. He chose to take advantage of the fact that he is self-employed and opted for "beach office" hours whenever he needed a nature fix. Old Travis was a meat-eater even though his body didn't like it. New Travis listened to what his body really craved and is now vegetarian. He was assessed with ADHD as an adult, and for many years he let it control him. Now, he says, "I run where my energy goes." He doesn't try to do it all, and he's done with being an accommodator.

A year or so after getting right with himself, he gained the courage to finally end his marriage. He was tired of trying to make something work that simply didn't, and he wanted more. Today, Travis's physical health continues to be a priority. He's got more energy and focus for the things that matter to him. At work, he's far more productive, his products are better, and his business has grown. He's more mindful with his kids and is in a new, healthy relationship. And he's happy.

Travis's story exemplifies how health and energy management can strengthen self-belief, clarify goals, and boost the discipline and focus needed to find success at higher levels.

Health as a Driver of Success

The human body is a machine like no other. In fact, your body is many different, interconnected machines functioning together to sustain you in all you do. Your heart, lungs, and other organs, your digestive system, musculature, and brain are individual machines within your body system that run at their own speed. But all operate systematically in relationship to one another to allow you to exist in this world.

Really, the human body is somewhat similar to the most complex human-made machines. The inner workings of your car, or dishwasher, or wall clock, for instance, consist of many individually functioning components that are all mechanically linked together to allow the machine to operate as it's meant to. There's nothing quite like the complexity of the human machine, though, and unlike man-made machines with rigid and inflexible parts, the numerous components that make up the human body are fluid and interconnected in ways that, unless you're a doctor or scientist, are largely beyond the realm of comprehension. The body just works, and we simply go about our lives driving this amazing human machine with little thought to the brilliance of its inner workings.

The moving parts in your car or the flywheels and cogwheels of the clock on the lunchroom wall are in rigid interrelationship, with little room for error. They either function together or they break. In that respect, the human body is an entirely different machine. Even with pretty sizable deviations from what would be considered normal, your body will still function and sustain meaningful life. You can forgo sleep and the body will still function. You can eat crappy food, drink too much alcohol or too little water, smoke cigarettes or other substances, and your machinery will remarkably keep operating. You can ignore the body's needs in so many small and large ways and—in the memorable words of the Timex watch ad from decades ago—it takes a licking and keeps on ticking. Probably more so than that clunky Timex.

If the machines of your body get taxed beyond their capacity, their breakdown usually manifests as fatigue or illness, sometimes fleeting, other times not. And yes, the machinery will eventually stop operating altogether, either through illness, accident, or old age. However, by tending to your human machine—in surprisingly simple ways, I'll note—you can boost your longevity and vastly improve the quality of your journey.

The wonderful truth about the human machine is that it is truly unlike any human-made machine in that instead of breaking down with use, it gets stronger, it works better, and it operates longer than if you didn't use it at all, at any age or stage of life. And when we use the body well and care for those internal mechanisms in the right ways, we vastly improve its external operations as well: creativity, critical thinking, problem solving, attention span, self-confidence, self-efficacy, social interactions, stress management, and more. Think about how much more productive, efficient, and enjoyable each day would be if these byproducts of good health were always operating near optimum. *Your body is an untapped storage house for higher levels of success.*

Here's another fascinating evolutionary truth about the human body that points to why movement in particular is so vital for brain function and creative output. Over two million years ago, in the time long before carriages or motor vehicles, even before horses were domesticated for use as transport, our early ancestors walked on average twelve to twenty miles per day to forage and hunt. A 2017 study by David Raichlen and Gene Alexander, published in *Trends in Neuroscience*, proposed that when humans shifted from a pseudo-sedentary, apelike existence to a more active hunter-gatherer existence, the jobs of foraging and hunting became much more physically and mentally demanding.[1]

At that point in history, foraging was a complex cognitive behavior. Our ancestors moved on foot through variable terrain without the aid of GPS. All day long. They used their memory not only to determine where to go, but also to remember how to get home. They had to pay attention to their surroundings, multitasking the entire time as they assessed the environment around them for food to eat, kept their eyes open for animals that could harm them, and traversed challenging terrain. As they moved, they constantly came across new predators, different dangers, and novel food sources and had to adapt. Along the way they developed rudimentary tools and built boats to assist their efforts. And so much of what they learned happened as they moved. This truth may explain how physical activity and the brain came to be so connected.

Our brains evolved while we were moving, not sitting, and yet here we are in the 21st-and-a-quarter century, brains and butts chained to our desks, sedentary, sloth-like, and stressed.

So much research supports the amazing benefits of health for productivity, happiness, and success, yet we ignore the truth because we have too much work piling up, too many tasks on our to-do list, too many distractions competing for our band-width, and no time or energy to get it all done. We mistreat the very machine that, when maintained properly, has unlimited capacity to transform how we work.

Counterintuitive to the power of stupid.

Every day we drive our sleep-deprived selves to work, then sit chained to a desk, staring at our monitor or phone screen for hours, devoid of any meaningful movement or social interac-tion. Our body sends us stress signals that we need a break, but instead we keep working. We ignore the nutritional and hydra-tion needs of our body, so energy drains, the mind becomes foggy, and we become productivity imposters. Working, sure, but nowhere near the level we're capable of. Such habits are functional in the short-term, but that's not how we should work. And it clearly runs counter to what science deems to be true. We're better when we move. We're better when we listen to the needs of our body. So, maybe it's time to do work differently?

Every thought you have, every movement you make or task you complete, every difficult problem you solve or burst of motivation you experience is driven from within your human machine. For peak physical, mental, emotional, and cognitive performance, the body you live in needs regular movement,

proper nourishment, hydration, social interaction, stress awareness, sleep, and relaxation. Every day. Sometimes several times
a day.

Nap Your Way to the Top

We've all been there: hunched at the keyboard, eyes
heavy, head bobbing, barely able to stay awake, and
wondering what to do. Here's a radical idea: take a nap.
Although sleeping on the job might seem like a risky
proposition, more and more big-name companies, such
as Samsung, Google, *HuffPost*, and Ben & Jerry's, promote short mid-shift naps by providing nap spaces in
their facilities, for employees' health, well-being, and
improved performance.[2] The benefits of a twenty-minute
nap include:

· Improved memory and information retention
· Increased relaxation
· Reduced depression and anxiety
· Increased energy

And if that's not enough to convince you, consider
NASA's groundbreaking 1995 nap study, which found
that a twenty-six-minute nap improves performance by
34 percent and alertness by 54 percent.[3]

Some experts suggest that anything beyond twenty
minutes is too long, as you risk falling into a deep sleep.
Jim Horne, former director of the Sleep Research Coun-
cil in the U.K., recommends a cup of coffee *before* you
nap. Since caffeine takes about twenty minutes to kick in,

you'll benefit from a short nap, then the coffee will rouse you and you'll feel more alert.

Don't have a nap room at your office? It wouldn't be the worst thing to put your head down on your desk for a ten-minute power nap. If you get caught in the act, lift your head, wipe the sleep from your eyes, and tell your boss or colleague, "I'm sleeping my way to the top... in a respectable way!"

Prioritizing Energy

Remember The Success-Energy Equation: $S = G \times f(B,D)^E$.

Success (S) equals clear goals (G), which will be achieved as a function (f) of the belief (B) you have in yourself regarding those goals, and the discipline (D) within you to do the work to achieve them.

When you factor energy management (E) into this formula, you'll reach for bigger goals, have a stronger mindset, and do excellent work. As you learn to prioritize specific energy management practices, you'll have a greater capacity to ignore the endless, prolific distractions of today's tech-connected world. You'll have more focus and discipline to do the work that really matters to you.

Attention to physical health will make you better at work and give you more energy for life. It will give you confidence, focus, and determination in everything you do. Yet, in our busy lives, health has become just another task on the to-do list. We attempt to squeeze in fitness and eat better to manage our weight or our blood pressure, but we ignore the other fascinating performance-based reasons to take care of our health. I mean, healthy weight and lower blood pressure are good, but a happy brain and ideas that are super-dialed in because of fired-up neural connections? Sexy! Really… do you come here often?

The hardiness of the human body is truly remarkable, so much so that it gives us a false sense of security regarding how much our human machine can actually endure. As we work, we regularly ignore the health and energy needs of our body and trick ourselves into thinking we're doing our best work. We're not. Your body knows better and it's amazingly resilient, but only to a point. You can't override how the body *actually* works. Eventually it will tell you so.

If success is important to you, energy matters. Doing great work is difficult if you're regularly running on empty. Your daily health and self-care must become a priority. Energy is the magic multiplier for success, and most people underestimate its power. Yes, health and self-care will give you physical energy and vitality, which we all need more of. I'll call that a side-benefit, though, because the true power that comes from energy management is the effect it has on your success mindset and your daily discipline.

When you have energy in the tank and feel good about yourself and your health, it changes how you approach most things. Self-efficacy—your belief in your ability to accomplish tasks—increases. As does self-esteem. Both of which lead to greater self-confidence with everything new and bold you choose to take on. And when belief in yourself is high, your mindset strengthens and, guess what, your discipline improves. You gain a greater work ethic for the goals you've set because you believe in your ability to crush them. You're more willing to do the freakin' work. Even if it's hard work. And it usually is. But you now have the focus, energy, and confidence to do whatever it takes. See how this works? Magic!

Wait, there's more! Once you heighten your mindset and discipline and begin to see results, you start to set bigger goals. And the goals scare you less because you now have a track record for success, *and* you have ample energy to fuel your efforts. You prioritize better, and you're less tempted by time-wasting distractions. You trust that you have the capacity to do the work.

In the chapters to come, we're going to unpack each of these success-energy variables, so you can understand how you work *now* and what it will take to help you perform *better* from now on. We'll explore the whys, hows, and what-not-to-dos of each variable, and you'll gain ideas and tools that will help you formulate your own powerful Success-Energy Equation.

Begin by becoming aware of where in your life you are on autopilot and ways to get present. Once you do, use that reignited awareness to reconnect with goals and plans that are meaningful to you, or create new ones.

Engage Your #SuccessEnergy: Health Habits

For good health, there are four health practices that should be a non-negotiable part of your daily routine. Sure, there are lots more creative and quick-fix ways to stay energized, but a busy schedule needs to get back to basics: move, eat, sleep, hydrate.

Move your body most days of the week at levels that challenge you. Your goal is to consistently do more than what is normal for you, with whatever you choose. A program that includes cardiovascular conditioning (walk, run, bike, swim) and strength training (weights, yoga) will provide good balance. And try to move more every day of the week.

Eat healthy most of the time. Consume less sugar and fewer processed foods, and more fruits and vegetables. Choose lean meats or try meatless options. Watch your portion sizes. Pack healthy snacks. It's not about giving up all the foods you love. It's about balance and mindfulness in how you fuel yourself.

Prioritize sleep as the restorative necessity that it is. Try for seven to nine hours of quality sleep, most days of the week. Create a healthy sleep environment that is cool, clean, and dark. Establish a pre-sleep routine that helps you wind down—hot tea, a warm bath, dim lights—and minimize activities that will turn your brain on. If you're prone to watching too much TV or playing digital games and the like, don't even turn them on, especially on the nights you're feeling particularly tired.

Hydrate throughout the day. Drink at least eight glasses of water (more if you're larger or active). The soda, juice, tea, or coffee you drink counts, but then you have to deal with the sugar and caffeine, so water is always best. If you feel tired, you may be dehydrated. If you regularly feel foggy in the afternoon, hydrate for energy and focus.

And reflect on these questions:

What are you already doing for your health that you are proud of?

What are some of the ways you would like to improve your health?

What small steps in each of these areas can you take today to move in the right direction?

Each day commit to making small steps to improve your movement, nutrition, sleep, and hydration. Consistency is key, and small steps count.

3

STUCK ON AUTOPILOT

---

66 The secret of your future is hidden in your daily routine. 99

MIKE MURDOCK

I F YOU WANT true success, it's vital that you know what that looks like for you, because if you don't know which direction you're going, it'll take a lot longer to get anywhere good. The first variable in The Success-Energy Equation—goals (G)—is about setting clear, exciting goals that you can't wait to tackle. Good goals help you clarify what you want out of work and life. That allows you to live closer to your purpose, and to be more conscious about the work you do so that it supports your goals and, ultimately, your success.

What do you want for yourself personally and professionally?

When you can answer that question with absolute clarity, and you can visualize the direction you're meant to go, the path to success will be much easier to travel. Despite this truth, busy people often find it challenging to clearly identify goals that matter to them. Goals are important, but the busyness of life steals away the time and presence necessary to clearly identify what we want.

When we're excessively busy, many of us navigate all or part of our lives on autopilot—making unconscious, automatic decisions that don't necessarily align with how we want to work and live—and that truth limits our success. Autopilot-living is a symptom of 21st-and-a-quarter-century stress. The day drones on as we check off to-dos without paying attention to whether we're doing the right work on the right tasks. We don't have the time or bandwidth to check in with ourselves.

You must have presence of mind when setting important goals. If you're on autopilot or have been in the past, you'll need to check in with yourself to make sure the path you're on aligns with what you aim to achieve. If you're off course, you're not alone. In a 2017 study by Mark Williamson and Renata Salecl, a whopping 96 percent of the three thousand people surveyed admitted they made decisions every day on autopilot.[1] That number may seem alarmingly high, but it's not surprising.

Human beings are creatures of habit; we're masters at creating routines so we can keep order and get things done. For instance, you likely follow the same order of operations each morning as you head into your day, perhaps some version of: brush your teeth, shower, dress (right sock first, then left), coffee, cereal, news on the iPad. And you probably need to pause right now to note the details of your *actual* routine, because it just happens every morning without you having to think about it. That systemization is your brain's way of project managing all it must process in a day.

It's said that the average adult makes about 35,000 remotely conscious decisions each day. If you exclude the seven hours when you're in decision-free slumber, that means you're making roughly two thousand decisions per waking hour, or one every two seconds. While that number may seem mind-blowingly high, it's not inconceivable if you consider that many of your decisions happen at the subconscious or semiconscious level.

You don't outwardly decide to scratch an itch, you just do it. You'll step around a pile of clothes on the floor or make space for a person entering an elevator without analyzing the necessity of those actions. You probably don't give much thought, if any, to the order of operations you follow as you sit down at your desk to work on your computer. But dozens of decisions are being made in a short time span: adjust chair just so, turn on computer, clear papers from line of sight, shift posture, choose pen from the jar, place it by notepad, prioritize to-dos in your mind, scratch itch, close door because there is noise in the hallway, put on sweater, sip coffee, turn notifications off on phone, glance at text messages as you do, open up email, delete, read, delete, delete, respond, and so on.

As you task-master your way through each day, whenever possible your brain will shift into automatic decision-making at the subconscious level—with simple tasks, rote skills, or anything that doesn't need your full attention—so it can save energy and free up your conscious mind to focus on more mentally challenging tasks.

As you walk to grab your morning coffee, you invariably navigate the hallway mindlessly, press the elevator button without thinking, make your way to your usual coffee shop without really paying attention; as you do all of this, your brain may be churning away on the work problem you left on your desk, or you might be staring at your device with no need to look where you're going as you figure out how to order lunch through your favorite restaurant's new online app.

Your ability to think about what *isn't* happening at any given moment is a cognitive triumph that helps your day run more smoothly. Until it doesn't. Autopilot is an evolutionary protection mechanism that stops our brain from overloading, but we're not meant to function in that mode for a long time. When autopilot becomes your go-to operating system, not just at work but in every aspect of your life, it's a sign that your system is overwhelmed, and 21st-and-a-quarter-century stress is creeping in. Left unchecked, it will impact your success, health, and happiness. And not in a good way.

Take Your Damn Break

When you're slammed, the idea of pausing to take a break feels impossible. There's only so much time to get it all done. But here's why you should take your damn break: on a busy day you will always run out of time, but with the right workday habits, you'll always have energy. Our bodies function on a rest-activity cycle called the ultradian rhythm. The term was coined by physiologist and sleep researcher Nathaniel Kleitman in the 1960s and was examined specifically in relation to our waking hours in the 1990s by Ernest Rossi. Throughout your workday you'll have three or four approximately ninety-minute periods of high productivity, when you're more alert and focused and get good work done. These times are usually interspersed with twenty-minute periods of fatigue, distraction, and sometimes drowsiness, when productivity dips.

Learn to recognize your productive times and take advantage of them to get great work done. And when that inevitable drop in energy shows up, take a break—even if you feel like you can't afford the time. If you always push through when your body needs downtime, you'll create more stress, which may lead to burnout, high blood pressure, ulcers, and weight gain. So, take your damn break:

· Leave your desk and go somewhere to relax, preferably where there is fresh air.
· Eat a healthy snack, walk, sit, and breathe.
· Talk with people you like.
· Go tech-free and give your brain the chance to re-oxygenate and recharge.

Research suggests that even a short, well-implemented break will offset boredom, increase creativity, and boost productivity upward of 20 to 40 percent.[2] That will more than make up for whatever you might have accomplished if you kept working through the fatigue.

Don't fight it. Work hard, yes... and if you want to do your very best every day, listen to your body and take twenty every ninety.

Twelve Signs You Are on Autopilot

Autopilot switches on automatically, and it can take a while before we're even aware that it's running our lives. You might be wondering then: *Am I stuck on autopilot?* Well, if you're feeling any level of overwhelm, busyness, distraction, or discontent in your life and any of the following scenarios resonate with you, the answer may be yes, and it could be time to start looking for the "off switch." Here are twelve signs you are on autopilot:

1. Your routine is predictable

You already know what you're doing next week (all week), who you'll talk to (same ten people), what you'll have for lunch (same as yesterday), even where you're going for holidays (same as last year), and it hasn't occurred to you to change things up. Life feels repetitive and there's no room for improvisation or last-minute changes.

We create routine to better manage stress and busyness, and that predictability saves us from having to make too many "unnecessary" decisions when our bandwidth is at capacity. But if you adhere too rigidly to those predictable routines, it can do more harm than shaking things up.

2. You don't look forward to the day ahead

You wake up and dread stepping into the day, because there's nothing exciting or inspiring to anticipate. You're not motivated to get on with it because you know what's going to happen. You can't understand why, out of nowhere, you no longer look forward to the day, because it wasn't always that way.

This sign is a byproduct of predictable routines. The routine we autopilot into, to manage the stress and busyness, is a blessing that eventually starts to feel like *Groundhog Day*, and it's hard to know how to reignite our drive once we lose it.

3. You start your day by checking your device

You wake up and your first entry point into the day is to check your phone. You tell yourself you're doing this to stay on top of things, but in reality it's an autopilot habit that takes control of your day from moment one. Then, throughout the day, your device is always within reach. You just checked it five minutes ago, but you feel the need to check it again right now, and to mindlessly scroll through emails and social media every chance you get.

This is a tricky one. Fatigue and busyness no doubt play into our device devotion, because when life is busy, connecting with the internet requires less energy than connecting with others. Rather than muster the energy to be present, we decompress with our devices until they become a source of distraction from doing our best work and then a dopamine-fed habit that is difficult to break.

4. You're stuck in your head

People are constantly jolting you back to the present because your mind often wanders or gets lost in deep thought. You tune out co-workers, your spouse, your kids, your dog, and you're not even aware you're ignoring them. It often feels like you're forgetting something. You are busy, distracted, or both.

> With so many things on our to-do lists, it's no wonder we're stuck in our heads. Executive functions in our brain's prefrontal cortex control short-sighted, reflexive behaviors so we can focus on planning, decision-making, problem solving, and the like. Our brain initiates autopilot so we don't forget to do all those important tasks. If the jobs don't get done, we get up into our heads until they're done, constantly thinking about what needs to be completed, or ruminating on what we didn't do or could have done better.

5. You do things without thinking

You act before considering whether the work you're tackling is the best use of your time, the right way to tackle it, or even if it's in your job description. Your goal is to get it all done, and you're so busy that you drone through the day just doing. It doesn't occur to you that you could be doing the wrong work, or someone else could be doing it for you. You never pause to reflect on how you're feeling or what you're doing.

> This is the epitome of autopilot. When there's a lot to do, we often put our heads down and plow through whatever comes our way. No time to prioritize or delegate. We can get it done in less time. This too becomes a habit that's hard to break.

6. You say yes without pause

When someone asks you for help, no matter what the ask, your default response is yes. You find yourself helping, hosting, volunteering, staying late, coming in early, or working on tasks that aren't in your job description or the least bit interesting to you. You let other people's agendas define your choices.

> It takes precious bandwidth to make decisions. Plus, we're busy anyway, so what's one more task? It may not be ours to do, but we get a sense of accomplishment, along with gratitude from those we help . . . which can be rewarding when we're stressed. Saying yes is also easier than delegating.

7. Your success-path feels stalled

You make a solid effort every day, but you don't seem to make worthwhile progress with your professional goals. You don't have the time or energy to contemplate let alone work on the goals that are important to you, and it's affecting your fulfillment on the job.

> When we work hard and don't achieve our goals, it feels baffling. But this happens partly because we do things without thinking and say yes without pause (see numbers 5 and 6). Working on too many of the wrong things will slow our path forward. Additionally, all that extra work eats up the spare time that could be used for the goals that matter most to us.

8. You procrastinate the good stuff

You never seem to have time or energy for fun, leisure, and personal growth. If you find a bit of time, you procrastinate and choose distractions over action. Your bandwidth is so overloaded it feels easier to zone out than to do activities you love.

> Refer back to point 7. When we're busy, we tend to prioritize work over fun. Otherwise, how else will we get it all done? That busyness leads to mental and physical fatigue, and it's hard to push ourselves to get out and get active or have fun

when we're tired and stressed. The Netflix binge is justified because we've been working so hard, right? Welcome to autopilot apathy.

9. You're not clear about what's important to you

You're busy and have a lot on your plate, yet you haven't taken the time to think about what's important to you in your work and life, or you don't really know. You go through each day making one unconscious decision after another and have lost sight of your dreams. You are not paying attention to what you need.

We do a lot of important things every day, so we are productive on one level, which justifies our flight paths... for a while. But the longer we operate on autopilot, the further we fly off course. It takes time and bandwidth to ponder possibilities, and when life is coming at us from all directions, karate chopping through the work is usually easier than slowing down and taking that personal and professional inventory.

10. You're always chasing time

You're often in a hurry, or running late, or you rush through tasks in front of you. You often feel time-crunched or up against deadlines and have surface interactions with the people around you. You often can't remember what you did throughout the day.

Time-chasing is a sign of autopilot because busyness breeds frenzy, and frenzy takes us out of the present. With lots to do, we move on to the next thing, and then the next, and with no breathing space in our schedules, of course we get backed up. Our brains will automate to avoid overload. Are you seeing a trend here?

11. You don't step outside your comfort zone

You can't remember when you tried something new or challenged yourself in a meaningful way. You feel like it's easier to stick with your routine, even if the routine is uninspiring.

> Competence requires less bandwidth than novelty. Every time we try something new our brain lights up and gets present to the fresh challenges and new skills to be learned. That requires energy, and since our schedules ensure we don't have any, we stick with what we know.

12. You feel stuck

You know that there's more to life than this, but you don't see a clear path forward. Life is too hectic, and you lack real energy to climb out of your rut.

> Number 12 sums up so many of those that precede it. "Stuckness" is a sign of autopilot because we feel it when we don't act on what matters most to us. To get more out of life, we must be present to it.

Autopilot Versus Awareness

How many of these twelve signs can you identify with? Whether all of them or just a few, be aware of the impact they may be having on your health, happiness, and success. Letting autopilot guide you through mundane activities, like driving to work or photocopying a stack of reports, is one thing, but you don't want it running the show when you've got important decisions to make or significant problems to solve—including the basic question about what you want for your life.

My coaching client Tara was a driven, smart, single woman with a leadership position in a growing company. She liked her work and it challenged her, but she was feeling uninspired and a bit burned out. She struggled with workday blahs and general malaise in everything she did, and it was affecting her productivity. She felt like a mouse in a maze, following the same predictable path to the cheese, and she was starting to resent the cheese. But since she really did value her work, we decided we'd explore the bigger picture of her routine.

Tara had a fifteen-minute walk to work that always began with a stop at the same coffee shop on the corner, where the baristas would have her usual order ready. She followed the exact same route to work, and landed at her desk pretty much on the dot of 7:45 a.m. Every day. She rarely took breaks, ate lunch at her desk, and often didn't leave the office until 6:30 p.m. She usually brought work home with her because she didn't have much of a social life.

Tara's routine presented a lot of areas to work on, but we started small with a shift in her morning plan.

Her first autopilot "shake-up" was simply to walk a different route to work every day for one week, and just notice. Sounds a bit simplistic and stupid, right? Maybe, but stay with me. Her route varied by only one or two blocks in either direction, but she discovered two new coffee shops, a quaint yoga studio, and a great little tucked-away sushi restaurant she had no idea existed. She realized that if she headed one block north, she had an unobstructed view of the mountains for part of her walk, and there was a lovely park she couldn't believe she'd never seen. Beautiful! And if she went two blocks in the other direction, there was a street lined with Japanese cherry trees, which made her look forward to spring. She noticed all sorts of other small and significant things along each new route that added interest and curiosity to what was previously a dull, predictable daily necessity.

Tara's new morning routine added a bit of time to her commute, but she arrived at the office refreshed, energized, and ready to tackle the day. She dubbed this walking commute her morning meditation and took great pleasure in tucking her phone away and walking with head up and eyes open. And then something really cool happened. She became curious about her neighborhood and life *beyond* work. She realized that while she loved her work, she spent far too much time there, and needed to get a life.

She popped into the yoga studio to see about classes, called a friend she hadn't seen in a while and invited her for sushi, and started to take lunch breaks out of the office a couple of days each week at one of the coffee shops she'd discovered. She also started taking more work breaks during the day and sometimes walked with some of her co-workers to the new park she'd spotted.

Over the course of several weeks Tara inched away from her predictable routine into a more fulfilling week that included variety and a little spontaneity. Not surprisingly, she began to work less, but her productivity and creativity improved. She felt more present and attentive to her work and surroundings and realized that she'd been on autopilot—making unconscious, automatic decisions that didn't align with how she wanted to work and live—for several years. She was glad to be back in control of her flight.

Who Controls Your Flight?

Autopilot is your brain's way of helping you work when so much around you isn't working. It's an immediately accessible solution to 21st-and-a-quarter-century stress, a survival mechanism that prevents your life from imploding. By automating a great deal of your daily processes, by not requiring you to be fully present to every demand on your precious bandwidth—no matter how busy and seemingly unmanageable life may get—your brain, and its autopilot feature, helps you navigate the chaos. The fascinating thing about autopilot is that it sneaks into your habits, and it can take a while before you realize it's messing with your success, because it rarely messes up your life. But that doesn't mean you should let it control the flight.

The phrase "going through the motions" describes it well. You're doing, but your heart and mind aren't fully in your tasks. You act out of habit and in a cursory way, without enthusiasm or real connection. On autopilot we become human robots who forget about goals and focus too much on task management. When this happens, we neglect health because we don't have the time or energy to fit it in. We let fatigue rule, and turn into productivity imposters. We lose sight of what's truly important to us in work and life.

As life flies at you from every direction day after day, you can keep doing what you've always done: square your shoulders and bulldoze your way through the chaos, flattening every last to-do until you're *too done*. But for how long? Or you can face the fact that some of that stuff you're chasing may be past its due date, or it's not yours to chase, or it used to be, but you'd rather be chasing different goals today, and you don't really know what those goals are.

How would it feel to be more in control of your day, to be more deliberate in the choices that carry you from morning to night, and for those choices to lead you toward greater health, happiness, and success?

If you're ready to go after meaningful, exciting goals, you must first get present to the routines and habits that may no longer be serving you. You must find that switch and shut off autopilot, even for a short while. You can't clarify and set truly meaningful goals if you're not fully present to what's in front of you right now. This first step—to shut off autopilot—will help you free up the energy and mental bandwidth that will be critical for what comes next. So, if you're ready to do the freakin' work, grab a pen or pencil and let's get started.

Engage Your #SuccessEnergy: Assessing Autopilot

Consider the degree to which you can relate to the following autopilot indicators by rating yourself on a scale of one to five, with one being *very true of me* and five being *not at all true of me*. Circle your response.

	Very true of me		Neither true or untrue		Not at all true of me
My daily routine is predictable.	1	2	3	4	5
I do not look forward to the day ahead.	1	2	3	4	5
I start my day by checking my device.	1	2	3	4	5
I cannot leave my device alone.	1	2	3	4	5
I am stuck in my head.	1	2	3	4	5
I do things without thinking.	1	2	3	4	5
I am not good at delegating.	1	2	3	4	5
I say yes without pause.	1	2	3	4	5
My success-path feels stalled.	1	2	3	4	5
I procrastinate the good stuff.	1	2	3	4	5
I do not have time or energy for fun/hobbies.	1	2	3	4	5
I do not know what is important to me.	1	2	3	4	5
I have not tried something new for a while.	1	2	3	4	5
I often run late.	1	2	3	4	5
I often feel time-crunched.	1	2	3	4	5
I feel stuck.	1	2	3	4	5

If you find yourself staring down multiple *one* and *two* responses, and you don't have the first clue how you got there, you flew in on autopilot. Take a closer look at each indicator and consider how often you find yourself in that space. All day, every day? Once or twice a day? Several times a week? How much is autopilot controlling your actions? Note that you don't have to be a full-time flyer to feel the negative effects of tuned-out living. You might see evidence of the signs only once or twice a day, but still they can hijack your mindfulness.

Additionally, you may have scored low on only a few indicators but the discomfort you feel because of them is weighing you down. If your success-path feels stalled, for instance, that truth can hang over you all day, every day, and it will affect your energy, mindset, and discipline. Let's dig a little deeper:

Which indicators trigger discomfort?

What emotions do you feel as you acknowledge that?

What feels heavy about each of the autopilot indicators that trigger you?

Which autopilot signs feel most urgent for you to address?

Which autopilot indicators can you change with simple awareness?

Do you see how answering these questions might help you start naturally shifting off autopilot, even for brief moments? The path to awareness takes practice, especially if you've been tuned out for a while. Be patient with yourself, and trust that with daily practice you can regain control of the flight.

4

FROM AUTOPILOT TO AWARENESS

“ Breathe: To pause. To make space.
To collect your thoughts. To remember.
To face the next moment. To choose. ”

KARM C.

ERHAPS YOU'VE HEARD this statement: "How you do anything is how you do everything." There's something to it, especially when it comes to how you set your pace for the day. This saying explains why Sunday morning feels so different from Monday morning. Sunday is the quintessential lazy, do-as-you-feel kind of day. You don't rush out of the gates: you might sit and read the news or listen to music over a drawn-out breakfast; you may decide in the moment what you'll do next, which in my household is sometimes not much. And even if you're rushing out the door to the mountains or to your kids' activities, there's a different energy connected to the pace, isn't there? Monday, on the other hand, has an urgency to it, a quickening that sets the tone for the day. Up and at 'em, check emails, breakfast on the fly, device always close at hand, go, go, go. How often does that Monday morning pace follow you through the entire week?

Twelve Ways to Move from Autopilot to Awareness

Now that you have a bit of awareness around the habits and behaviors that switch you into autopilot, let's take a closer look at ways to regain control of your daily flight. Reaching your goals will be more difficult if you have no idea which direction you're flying. Once you know, though, you'll find it much easier to focus on the goals and plans that hold true meaning for you. You'll clarify the direction in which you're meant to go. Let's consider twelve ways to shift from autopilot to awareness.

1. Wake up mindfully

After your alarm rings, give yourself a few minutes to just lie in bed and breathe. Check in with yourself before you check in with the world. How did you sleep? How does your body feel? How about your mind? What feels good about this day? What can you look forward to? What do you need for yourself at the start of this day? This simple ritual is a powerful way to begin the day on your terms. So often, the first thing we do once the alarm rings is reach for the phone plugged in at our bedside, and within moments of gaining consciousness we're checking email or scrolling our social channels. If that's you, can you stop doing that? Instead, try these two tips to delay that shift into autopilot:

Make your bedroom a no-phone zone

There are only two things that should take place in that room, and TV and phones aren't on the list (wink, wink). Buy a good old-fashioned alarm clock and leave your phone in the kitchen.

Delay that first check-in

If you must have your phone at your bedside, delay laying eyes on it until you mindfully check in with yourself. You've just gone through all those sleeping hours without looking. Surely you can gift yourself fifteen additional minutes of tech-free mindfulness?

2. Set intentions at the start of your workday

As you lie in bed, don't just whine in your head about how tired you are. Think about what you'd like to accomplish during the day. Think about what will help you feel successful. Decide how you want to feel at the end of the day. You get to choose. Autopilot doesn't have to take over.

Then, before you begin your workday, take five minutes to write down three objectives you absolutely want to complete by the end of the day. My list usually includes two or three work-related tasks and one personal goal, often to do with exercise or self-care. Once I make my list, I start on the first work-related goal, sometimes before even checking email.

When you set your intentions, you take back power over your schedule. You decide where you want to focus your energy. You give yourself permission to set aside other people's requests and prioritize your own work first. You'll have plenty of time in your day to address other people's needs, so start with your own and let that "take-control" mentality carry you into your day.

3. Shake up your daily routine

This simple tip is such an effective way to move from autopilot to awareness, as we saw with Tara's morning walk to work in the previous chapter. When life is busy, we automate everyday happenings to free up bandwidth, but in the process, life becomes mundane.

So, shake it up. Sit in a different spot at the breakfast table and change what you eat. Drive a different route to work or ride your bike instead. Check out a different coffee shop or skip the coffee and try a walk outdoors instead. If you normally eat your lunch at your desk, head to the lunchroom or a nearby park. Invite someone new to join you. Embrace little changes.

Decide on a simple shake-up, then notice how your brain lights up to help you do things differently. It's switching off autopilot, and that's a good thing. When your brain has to work, you have to be present. Try a different shake-up every day. Have some fun with it. Pay attention to what you've been missing.

4. Try something new

How long has it been since you've tried something new, something you've *never* done, or something you haven't done in a really long time? When life gets busy, we become creatures of habit, and tend to gravitate toward activities that we're good at. Competence requires less bandwidth, after all, but it also draws us into autopilot.

When you step outside that comfort zone by trying something new, your brain and body fire up in ways that keep you present. I'm a competent mountain biker on some pretty gnarly terrain, but my first time on a stand-up paddleboard on glass-like water was a wobbly, foot-clenching, mind-racing exercise in staying upright. Which I didn't. And I loved the newness and challenge of it. I got excited about getting better at it, which made me want to try it again.

Learning happens when you stretch beyond your comfort zone. Try something new. Embrace a new physical activity or sign up for an evening art or cooking class. Try out a different fitness class or weight routine at your gym. Get involved with a corporate challenge at work or say yes to a project that will stretch you a bit.

It's OK to not be good at everything; in fact, novelty strengthens brain and body in a way that competence can't. The next time someone asks you, "What's new?" wouldn't it be fun to have an interesting answer?

5. Detox from your device

Anyone who has ever destroyed or lost their phone, or left it somewhere by accident, knows that gut-clenching feeling of "Oh my God, what will I do without it?" In an interview with the *Guardian*, former Apple programmer Chris Marcellino, who helped develop the iPhone's push notifications, stated that smartphones hook people by engaging the same neural pathways as gambling and addiction. Some even suggest that designers are exploiting that truth for their own financial gain.[1]

Most social media platforms, games, and apps that you check in with regularly are designed with features that draw you in, again and again—gamification, likes, comments, pop-up news stories. When your brain taps into fresh knowledge or expects a reward, it triggers the release of the feel-good neuro-transmitter dopamine. When we need a dose of "comfort or calm" we pull out the phone to get another hit. We're addicted to our devices, so much so that being separated from the little wonders can cause twitches akin to withdrawal . . . maybe it *is* withdrawal? Smartphone addiction creates a vicious cycle of cortisol-fed stress response versus dopamine-driven calming that we repeat all day long:

> You wake up in the morning and check your phone (dopamine); you see all the emails that came in overnight, and a text from your boss (cortisol). You scroll through Instagram over breakfast (dopamine, dopamine, dopamine), so now you're late and you have to rush (cortisol), and you're driving so you can't respond to the alerts that are coming in (cortisol), but as soon as you pull into your parking spot you pull out your phone and see what you missed (dopamine). You've got a meeting first thing and you try not to check your phone (cortisol), but you sneak a quick peek here and there (dopamine), and when you return to your desk, you update yourself on emails, texts, and social channels, and you feel good (dopamine). Except about that one snarky post from your so-called friend (unfriend, cortisol). You get to work on the day's tasks and progress well (also dopamine), but then you take a procrastination break, and the guilt of it causes you stress (cortisol), but only until you feel the smooth screen of your phone under your thumb, and swipe (dopamine) and open up the app, game, or social channel (dopamine, dopamine).

Our brains are tired of it.

The dysfunctional relationship we have with our devices is making us dumb and anti-social. Plus, they're one of the biggest contributors to autopilot *and* 21st-and-a-quarter-century stress, so why not distance yourself from your device at strategic points during your day or week? Here are a few ideas:

· Leave your phone at your desk when you take a break. Walk outdoors, read a book with pages you have to turn. Talk face-to-face with a colleague.

· Don't take your phone with you to work meetings, and instead allow yourself to be fully present. In fact, make phone-free meetings an office policy and see how much more efficient your meetings will be.

· Leave your phone in the glove box of your car when you meet someone for coffee or lunch. There's nothing more irritating or disrespectful than visiting a friend who is constantly checking their device. Don't be that person.

· When you arrive home after work, park that device from the moment you park your car. Enter your home with full awareness of the people waiting to see you and give them at least fifteen minutes of your undivided attention.

· Go 100 percent tech-free during family meals. Enjoy real social interaction with your family and show your loved ones that they're valued more than whatever is on your screens.

· Turn Saturday afternoons into tech-free social time. Have fun outside, read hard-copy books, play board games, explore your neighborhood, go out for lunch.

· Stop all online interactions every day from 8 p.m. onward. Physically shut down your device when you do, and don't turn it on again until the next day... after a bit of morning mindfulness.

Or, if these ideas scare you, start smaller:

- If one app, site, or game is particularly distracting, restrict its use for a few days.
- Take a break from one of your social media channels.
- Delete certain apps from your device to help the detox.

Digital distraction is a growing problem that, for many, will require practice and a commitment to change akin to giving up smoking. If you want to get present to life, try it—even in short bouts. When you decide to take a digital pause, it's not enough, however, to turn your phone facedown on the table next to you. The fact that you can still see it means your attention is being hijacked. Studies have shown that if your phone is visible, it will remain an ongoing source of distraction that will hamper your ability to connect to the person or task in front of you.[2] Your purse or pocket is only slightly better. If you can, leave your device in another room, or in a desk drawer. If the idea of that makes you twitch, then you should double down your efforts to make it happen.

Hey Google, I Don't Need My Phone

As I researched this book and the pervasiveness of digital distractions and 21st-and-a-quarter-century stress, it occurred to me that, like many people, I often pick up my phone to google something important (or not) and then get lured into social media or other such mindless time wasters simply because I have my phone in my hand. So, I decided to invest in a Google Home voice assistant as an experiment in disconnecting. Strange, right? Hear me out.

The device sits on my kitchen table, where I can ask it anything from the news to the weather to how many ounces are in a cup. Instead of picking up my phone to find the answer to a question, I can simply ask: "Hey Google, is white noise or pink noise better for sleep?" I get a simple answer (both are good, but pink seems to be slightly better for promoting deep sleep) and avoid getting sucked into the endless mindlessness that is my smartphone. I find that once the workday is done, I put my phone on its charging pad and pick it up far less than I used to.

If you find that you're tethered to your smartphone day and night and you need practice letting go, consider the use of voice assistant technology to help you disconnect. It's an unconventional solution, but it's working for me.

6. Connect with those around you

In an age of device addiction and distraction, we take human interaction for granted. When you connect meaningfully with someone, an energy exchange occurs that helps you become present. Whether you engage more openly with the barista at the coffee shop, connect with a good friend over lunch, or simply ask someone for help, those human interactions have a way of bringing you into the moment. They're also good for your health and well-being.

A study published in *Science* magazine in 1988 showed that a lack of social connections may be more harmful to your health than obesity, smoking, or high blood pressure.[3] Social connections strengthen the immune system and lower inflammation. Back in 1988 we didn't have devices to draw us further from those interactions, so this study may be even more relevant today. In 2018, former British prime minister Theresa May appointed a minister for loneliness to help tackle problems associated with social isolation.[4] A study by the British government uncovered a worryingly high rate of loneliness among seniors and marginalized people across all ages and recognized that social isolation can have serious repercussions on a person's mental health and mortality.[5]

We are social animals by nature, and when we don't connect with others regularly, we feel less happy, and experience higher rates of loneliness, anxiety, and depression. Plus, isolation leads to more isolation. Without those connections we're likely to withdraw even more, which leads to further isolation and a higher likelihood of experiencing the negative effects of it.[6] And, by the way, connecting on social media doesn't count. That kind of "connecting" has been known to increase anxiety and depression. You can cultivate meaningful connections with friends and strangers alike when you:

- Are social with people you like and plan special time with people you love.

- Accept help when it's offered or ask for it when you need it.

- Learn about someone and explore things you have in common.

- Are open to emotional support when you're in a tough spot, or advice when you're stuck.

- Engage in eye-to-eye conversations that balance listening and sharing.

- Talk on the phone with friends and family who are separated by distance.

- Be curious and ask questions of people you want to know better. Listen for the answers.

- Do fun, laughter-inducing activities with other people.

Whom do you connect with regularly, and do those interactions fill you up and provide support? If they do, work hard to maintain the strength of those relationships. And if they don't, step outside your comfort zone to cultivate new, more meaningful connections.

7. Get outside

You know how good it feels to be in nature. I hope you do, anyway. The sounds of the forest or ocean, the scent of the earth and everything that grows, the beauty of the mountains, trees, water, sunshine, the fresh air. When we spend time in nature, stress abates, we forget our worries, we think more clearly and perhaps more creatively. In an increasingly demanding world, time in nature can improve mood, boost energy, and help us re-center.

Being with Mother Nature, breathing in all her sights and smells, is the best way to become alive to the present moment; for many, though, it's a rare occurrence, so much so that there's a name for the lack of it. "Nature-deficit disorder" (NDD), although not a recognized condition yet, was coined by journalist and author Richard Louv in his book *Last Child in the Woods*.[7] Louv argues that all of us, especially children, are spending more time indoors, becoming alienated from nature and more vulnerable to negative moods or reduced attention span. Causes include loss of open space, busy schedules, and digital distraction. Louv says that NDD affects "health, spiritual well-being, and many other areas, including [people's] ability to feel ultimately alive."

Perhaps this deficit has fueled the forest bathing movement. Based on the Japanese *shinrin-yoku* (*shinrin* meaning "forest," *yoku* meaning "bath"), forest bathing—also known as forest therapy—is essentially a slow, mindful walk through the woods, bathing in the atmosphere and taking in the forest through our senses.

You may be thinking, *Who has time for a trip to the forest?* Fair enough: if your busy, city-focused life is low on forest visits, connect with nature where you can find it. Qing Li, author of *Forest Bathing: How Trees Can Help You Find Health and Happiness*, says even small connections with nature—with a tree or patch of grass in an urban park, for instance—can have a profound effect on well-being.[8] So, if you're feeling the effects of autopilot, head outdoors, find some green grass to wiggle your toes in or a tree to sit under, and tune in to Mother Nature. Sit and breathe her in, notice her beauty, pay attention to her sounds. She has a way of drawing us into the here and now when technology has pulled us away from it.

8. Get moving

The benefits of physical exercise are numerous, but perhaps one of the most profound in this day and age is its ability to help us increase focus—in the moment and for hours afterward.

When I mountain bike on a speedy section of single-track, in order to stay upright and away from obstructions I have to be fully in the moment and pay attention to my surroundings as I maneuver my bike along the trail. I must notice and navigate the roots and rocks on the path, and the trees I'm whizzing by. When I mountain bike, my mind is unlikely to be distracted by work issues, and I'm certainly not looking at my phone. After I ride, I always feel more mentally alert.

In his book *Brain Rules: 12 Principles for Surviving and Thriving at Work, Home, and School,* John Medina cites research that suggests exercisers outperform non-exercisers on tests that measure long-term memory, reasoning, attention span, and problem solving.[9] It stands to reason that, if you have important work that needs your full attention, planning at least thirty minutes of cardiovascular movement ahead of that work would be beneficial, as would scheduling regular movement throughout the week. Consider the types of activities you enjoy. Whether you walk, run, bike, dance, indoor climb, ski, skate, golf, swim, dig in the garden, or chop wood, those activities don't work well on autopilot. Purposeful movement requires your presence of mind.

The more challenging the activity, the less chance you have of mind-wandering. So, if you engage in simpler activities like walking or running, try doing them without music plugged into your ears. Experiment with just being in the moment with your activities. Listen to your body, pay attention to your surroundings, and savor the feeling of purposeful movement.

9. Clear the clutter

When you autopilot through life, it's easy to let your surroundings become disorganized and messy. You don't pay attention to where you put things, or you use something and don't take time to put it away when you're done. At work you might file papers in the wrong spot or let them pile up on your desk. At home you might mindlessly toss your keys and wallet on the counter, discard your jacket and shoes without thinking, or search endlessly for something lost in a stack of other misplaced items. All that distracting clutter will lock you in autopilot.

There's something wildly satisfying about tidying. I'm not suggesting you become a professional feng shui practitioner or learn how to "spark joy" with Marie Kondo and her KonMari revolution (although she seems to be onto something). But even a simple clutter-clearing in the spaces where you spend a lot of time—office, kitchen, living room, bedroom—will help you feel calmer and more present in your surroundings. To clear clutter, you must wake up to the mess. You have to go through belongings to decide their importance; pause long enough to connect with the items you're tidying so you can decide if you will keep, file, or toss whatever is in your hand. It takes a bit of time, but the effort is worth it.

Begin where you spend the most time. If you work full time, your workspace might need sprucing up. If you're a stay-at-home parent, your kitchen or living room might need organizing. And yes, if you spend long days in your vehicle, you'll feel better if it's clean and tidy too. Don't overthink this one. Set a timer for twenty minutes and do what you can with the space you're in. Even a short bout of tidying can declutter mind and spirit, and help you be more present to your surroundings.

10. Get making

I once had a client who de-stressed by putting together big, thousand-piece puzzles. It's not my idea of de-stressing, but for him it was a meditative practice that helped him slow down and be in the moment. I have a couple of friends who like to knit when they have spare time, a few others who paint (pictures, not walls), and others who tie fishing flies for fun, fix bikes for friends, or make their own jewelry. In the spring and summer, I like to dig my hands in the dirt and make my garden come to life. You might play an instrument or build model airplanes or bake wonderful cookies and cakes or build things in your garage. When we "make," we're in the moment. We get drawn into the task at hand, and slow down to the pace of whatever it is we're making.

Are there such activities in your life that might need resurrecting? Is there a creative endeavor you'd like to try? If you have no idea where to begin, keep it simple. Buy an adult coloring book and new colored pencils and have fun revisiting your childhood. Grab a pen and paper and doodle whatever comes to mind. It's amazing how, in the act of making, we can bring more presence to life's little pleasures.

11. Do fewer waste activities per week

"Waste" activities are those we engage in throughout the day that won't help us get ahead personally or professionally, and in this technology-driven world we've got lots of them: mindless television, online games, social media, non-work-related internet, scrolling endlessly. A waste activity can also be time spent with people who don't fill you up, or a meeting that doesn't get you anywhere, or anything that makes you think, *I should do something better with my time.*

If you usually scroll mindlessly through social media during your lunch break, choose a tech-free lunch and read a book instead, or go for a walk. If you often binge-watch Netflix in the evenings, replace some of that screen time with a more worthwhile activity. On autopilot, your default downtime behaviors will more often than not gravitate toward waste activities that allow you to numb out. And although we all need moments to sit and stare into space (or at the television), too much of that will keep you stuck.

12. Just breathe

This tip may be the simplest and most underused way to get off autopilot, which is baffling because it takes literally seconds to fill your lungs (right to the bottom) with energizing oxygen. Yet it's as though in the busyness of life we tell ourselves we don't have time for a full breath. Then we stressfully breathe into the top third of our lungs and miss out on the meditative influence of slow, deep breathing. Here's the thing: your body knows how to breathe. Breathing is a vital bodily function that your reptilian brain controls, so we just let it happen behind the scenes and forget to take it off default. Yes, our breathing operates on autopilot, which is probably a good thing because, with all we have going on, we'd otherwise forget to do it. But when you take your breathing off default and mindfully guide yourself through even four deep, cleansing breaths of air, the benefits are twofold. First, you immediately feel the energizing effect of oxygen as it fully enters your body. It feels different from default breathing, more purposeful and cleansing. Second, if you allow yourself to sit and breathe like this for even two minutes, you give yourself the chance to shut off autopilot, to become present, and to let your body and mind pause long enough to tell you what they need. And it's likely *not* to go back on autopilot.

Give yourself short breathing breaks throughout the day. Set a timer to alert you every ninety minutes, then stop what you're doing and breathe slowly and deeply for a couple of minutes. For a more in-depth description of this tip, read the #SuccessEnergy section at the end of this chapter, then schedule in your breathing breaks.

PRESENCE TAKES practice, so decide how you will practice getting off autopilot. Here's an idea: make waking up mindfully and setting your intentions at the start of your workday non-negotiables. These two practices alone can be transformational. Buy that alarm clock and remove that phone from your bedroom, check in with yourself before you check in with the world, and set your intentions for the day before your inbox hijacks your plans. From there, any time you sense that you're operating on autopilot, try another of the tactics above to get present.

Engage Your #SuccessEnergy: Two-Minute Time-Out

If you're busy, stretched, and stressed you may fight this practice. Please don't. Any time you begin to feel out of sorts, unfulfilled, or disconnected, one simple, powerful action will aid your shift from autopilot to awareness. In the busyness of your life it may not occur to you that it's an option. Yet it's readily available to you at a moment's notice, if you decide you need it: stop, pause, breathe. Slow the heck down. Create space to pay attention. Take a two-minute time-out. Nothing better helps you reconnect to here and now.

Pick up the device that is no doubt in arm's reach and set a timer for two minutes. Press start, then sit, breathe, and notice. Your eyes can be open or closed. You can focus on your breath, your heartbeat, where you're holding tension in your body… or on nothing. Breathe in through your nose for four seconds, pause for a second, then exhale out your mouth for four seconds. Do this for just two minutes.

The only expectation for this two-minute time-out is that you try it. Do it now. I'll wait…

IF LIFE is bearing down on you like a charging bull, it may feel counterintuitive to sit in one spot for fifteen seconds, let alone two minutes. You might get run over. But when you press on the brakes, you shut off autopilot. So, become aware of your pace and breathe—for just two minutes—then notice what's here right now.

Busy people often feel uncomfortable with stillness, perhaps because when there's lots to do, a pause of any appreciable length seems like a frivolous waste of valuable time. When we pause, it's like the brain can't comprehend—given the mountain of work we're staring down—that we *chose* to do it. To get us going again, it sends messages to the body to fire it up. As we sit, we feel restless or fidgety and unable to clear work-related thoughts from our head, so before long we abandon the breath and go back to tackling the task list. These moments of awkward pause, as with anything that you're not good at, have to be practiced until you get better at them.

If you're a human doing, you must practice becoming a human *being*.

This two-minute time-out is short enough that you shouldn't feel excessive discomfort, and long enough for you to experience the power of pause. It's short enough that you can do it several times a day as the need arises—when stress is mounting, when you feel overwhelmed by something or someone, when you just need to slow down and gather your thoughts—and long enough to allow your heart rate and breath to level off, and create a bit of calm.

PART II

READY, SET, GOALS

5

GOOD GOALS, GREAT GAINS

" If you don't know where you are going,
you might wind up someplace else. "

YOGI BERRA

AS YOU BECOME more present in your life, something amazing starts to happen. You begin to want something more... different... better for yourself. As you pay genuine attention to your work, the people in your life, your activities, how you use your time, and how all of it makes you feel, you might find yourself pondering questions like, *What now, what next, what do I really want for myself?*

In The Success-Energy Equation—$S = G \times f(B,D)^E$—the first variable delves into these very questions. In the formula, the path to success (S) begins with good goals (G). Goal clarity is vital for higher levels of success at anything. As the epigraph at the beginning of this chapter suggests, if you're unclear about where you're going, you're bound to end up somewhere you don't want to be.

Goal setting is a powerful way to clarify where to focus your time and energy. Whether you love goals, hate them, set then forget them, or fully embrace them, done correctly they can be a game-changer. Hopefully you embrace goals as the direction clarifying tool that they can be, but if you're like most people I speak to, you probably don't love them. In the busyness of life, there may be a good reason for that.

Goal Setting and
21st-and-a-Quarter-Century Stress

To set worthwhile, energizing goals that you're excited to tackle, you need to know where you are in your life right now—good, bad, or in between—and have some sense of how you'd like to improve or change it. You need time to craft goals that will help you get there, and, of course, energy to do the work. If you autopilot through each day in the throes of 21st-and-a-quarter-century stress, goals will be the last thing you want to tackle.

Think about the mental, physical, and emotional fatigue that you feel at the end of a busy, stressful day, then add to that the burden of the constant digital noise that has been vying for your attention too. You may have goals you really value, but under these circumstances you will no doubt struggle to find the time or energy to chase them. For many of us it's probably accurate to say we fail to make the time, perhaps because we give too much of it to our device, or to other distractions and low-priority tasks.

The distraction that is prevalent with 21st-and-a-quarter-century stress means you spend more time with your device and less time with your thoughts. You connect to the internet and disconnect from what you truly want and need for yourself. Your goals become murky, and you don't make the time to clarify them. Additionally, that digital connectedness allows you to see what everyone else is doing in their lives, and "comparisonitis" may kick in. You observe what friends, family, and colleagues post about their work and life and you begin to question your own path: *Do I need to do more? Should I be approaching things differently? Are my goals good enough?* In an effort to keep up with the Joneses you may feel overwhelmed, or adjust your plans, or default to inaction. But as you flip the switch on autopilot and become more present to everything happening in your life and the real world—with work, family, friends, your health—you may begin to view goals and goal setting in a more favorable light.

Why Goals Matter (Now More Than Ever)

If there's one good reason to get behind goal setting, it's this: 21st-and-a-quarter-century stress and all the digital distractions, global chaos, and overall busyness that are part of it mean that if you truly want to get things done, focus and clarity matter now more than ever.

When you set a goal, your attention is naturally drawn toward what you should do next. Your brain starts to look for ways to accomplish that goal and you gain focus, which is an antidote to all the distractions and low-priority tasks that compete for your attention every day. If you maintain that focus long enough to see progress, you'll gain momentum. Progress is addicting. As you make headway on that goal, your brain rewards you with a hit of dopamine, which inspires you to keep at it so you can continue to feel those good feelings. Momentum is a powerful motivator.

Goals also provide a touchstone for what you should say yes and no to throughout your day. When faced with decisions about how to allocate your time, you can ask yourself, *Will this task help drive my goals?* If it won't, you'll have a good reason to say no. Let's face it, most of us know what it feels like to spend time on tasks that are misaligned with our goals. Doing so is frustrating because it slows progress. Success requires deliberate action on the tasks that will help you achieve your goals, so what you say yes to matters.

You may find it difficult to say no to work tasks, even if they don't align with your goals and especially if they've been mandated by others. When this happens, first, do your job. Sometimes we have to do work that we don't love to get to the work that we do. If it happens often, it may be a sign you need to rethink the job you're doing, or at the very least negotiate the types of tasks that make up your job description.

Achieving your goals strengthens self-efficacy, your belief in your ability to accomplish a task. Every action that drives you forward will remind you that you're capable and shape you into the type of person who *can* achieve goals. It all sounds convincing, but goal setting still gets a bad rap because so many people set goals they never achieve. Goals fail for a lot of reasons, the most common being a lack of clarity about them, underestimating their size or difficulty, juggling too many priorities while chasing the goal, bad timing, and having no clear plan for execution.

Five Facets of Good Goals

I want you to keep the process of goal setting simple, but there are a few things to consider if you want to create good goals that aren't merely "set and forget." Consider these five pointers as you sit down to craft your goals.

1. Size matters

In their 1994 book *Built to Last: Successful Habits of Visionary Companies*, Jim Collins and Jerry Porras introduced the concept of Big, Hairy, Audacious Goals, or BHAGs, which are long-term goals that everyone in a company can understand and rally behind.[1] While it's good to think big and set lofty goals, for many people the idea of "big, hairy, and audacious" feels more like "big, *scary*, and *I can't do this*." And if the size of the goal overwhelms you with fear, you'll freeze and avoid the work.

Setting a goal that scares and challenges you just the right amount is important. If it doesn't feel a bit edgy, the goal's probably not big enough. Every goal should pull you outside that comfort zone enough to help you grow. So, here's where size matters. It's great to dream big, but when it comes to execution, it's OK to start small.

If the goal you set is so big that you can't comprehend when and how you'll achieve it, don't abandon it. Instead, break it down into chunks that you can more easily manage in shorter time frames. A goal that can be realized in six to twelve weeks will be easier to stick with than one that won't bear fruit for several months or years. Once you've accomplished one part of the goal, set your sights on the next phase.

My friend Martin Parnell is an ultramarathoner, which means he regularly runs races that are fifty to one hundred miles in distance. The very thought of running for fourteen hours or more in one go is, to me, scary and crazy. Interestingly, at first, it was for Martin as well. So were regular marathons before he trained to that distance. So were short runs before that. Martin wasn't even a runner until his mid-forties, when he was challenged to run the 2003 Calgary Marathon with two of his brothers. He had five months to train, and since he was essentially starting from zero, his first goals were to run five- and ten-kilometer races, then a half-marathon, right on up to full marathon distance.

That first marathon fired up a love of running in Martin that would evolve into ultramarathons, ironman triathlons, and an extraordinary goal he called "Marathon Quest."[2] In 2010, seven years after he became a runner, Martin set a goal to run 250 marathons in one calendar year to raise $250,000 for Right to Play, an international organization that, through play, teaches disadvantaged children valuable leadership skills. His Marathon Quest began on January 1 of that year with the plan to run five marathons per week for the entire year. I won't go into the details of the quest, but I will say that, because of sound planning, training, and support—and a whole bunch of grit—Martin accomplished his goal, and raised over \$320,000 for Right to Play, with more money to come after the quest was done.

Every big goal that Martin set for himself, he broke down into chunks that his mind and body could manage at the time. Each small success led to the completion of another part of his bigger goal, and when he conquered that bigger goal, he'd set another that was just out of his reach.

The goals you set for yourself might not be as crazy and colossal as Martin's, but whatever their size, they're important, and you'll increase your chances of crushing them if you break them down and "go small."

2. Be personal *and* professional

When you set goals for yourself, do you tend to focus on personal goals or professional ones? Or do you give attention to both? If you want to effectively balance your time, energy, and outcomes, it's essential to get personal *and* professional with your goals.

Although that makes sense in theory, many people I speak to prefer to focus on professional over personal goals. Perhaps it's because, in our work-driven lives, those professional goals—the promotion, the business idea, the new product, the MBA—will drive financial security and ultimate success, so we put our goal-setting energy there. It's also true that many companies require employees to set quarterly and annual goals, so in essence we're forced to set professional goals. Or maybe we value personal goals, but they take a back seat because after pursuing those professional goals we run out of time or energy. When work stress is high and fatigue rules, the last thing we want to do outside of work is more work. When we work on those personal goals, however, quality of life improves in meaningful ways. Personal goals provide much-needed balance—a focus on health, loved ones, and leisure that helps us restore and refocus. We often underestimate the power of personal goals, but they give us purpose beyond work, and when work gets tough, personal goals help us lighten up about it.

In what ways do you want to advance your career growth? What personal goals do you have that will improve your health, happiness, and success? Personal and professional goals are inextricably linked. They feed each other and drive success at everything.

3. Put it in writing

I can't tell you how many people I've surveyed who say they hate writing down their goals. In my audiences, easily 75 percent of any room will reluctantly admit they don't like to write down their goals. In workshops that I lead, I regularly have to prompt people to put pen to paper, and the pushback I get is remarkable. But not surprising.

Most people avoid writing down their goals because doing so makes the goal more real. Once we write it down, we need to do something about it, which requires work. And if we don't do the work (as has happened on many occasions in the past) we meet with feelings of guilt and failure (yet again). And God forbid anyone should *see* that goal, because then they will ask about it, or try to hold us accountable . . . which will add to those feelings of guilt and failure. So, to avoid all that, we simply bypass writing down our goals. Can you relate?

When you write down your goals—especially when you write them well—you extract them from your subconscious and fire up your gray matter to work on achieving them. Yes, you'll have work to do, but if you set a worthwhile goal, don't you want to achieve it?

Here is the science-based reason for pondering options and putting pen to paper: the act of contemplation alerts your brain to seek out the goals and dreams you've awakened to. When you write those goals down, it helps your brain embed that information for ongoing access. As you think about what you want for yourself, a biological process called "encoding" transports that information to the brain's hippocampus, where it's analyzed. From there, the brain decides whether to store that goal in long-term memory or discard it. Coined the "generation effect" by neuropsychologists, this principle suggests that people have better memory for thoughts and ideas they've generated themselves than for ones they've merely read. Your ideas and what you want for yourself matter. But your brain needs about nine to twenty seconds to embed those ideas in long-term memory.

When you think about what you want and visualize what it will look and feel like, you begin that process. Then, when you write it down, you get to access the generation effect again, and you vastly increase the chances of that goal being embedded in your memory. No matter how big or small the goal, or how long it will take, your brain—in a bid to seek pleasure and avoid discomfort—sets out to accomplish that goal. As you navigate your day, you'll begin to notice people, opportunities, and pathways that can bring you closer to what you want.

Let's say you want to go after your executive MBA. You don't know much about the process, but you know it will be good for career growth. You visualize how that degree will open doors. It excites you, so you write down the goal and commit to learning more. The seed has been planted.

That day, as you walk to grab a coffee, a billboard you've walked by dozens of times suddenly catches your eye: QUEEN'S UNIVERSITY EXECUTIVE MBA PROGRAM. When you head home at the end of the day, you overhear two people in the elevator talking about the pros and cons of another popular MBA program and why online may not be the way to go. You don't usually tune in to other people's conversations, but you heard *that*.

That evening an ad on TV attracts your attention. It's for yet another MBA program. Suddenly you see signs everywhere. Crazy? Not really. Chances are those signs were always there, and you didn't notice them until your brain switched on to seeing them. Remember, your brain wants you to accomplish that goal, and it will alert you to information that will increase your chances of success. So, clarify what you want. Write that stuff down. And for an extra boost, follow the next tip.

4. Put it where you can see it

If you want to add fire to that pen and paper goal, put that piece of paper where you can see it regularly, where you can read it and be reminded of what you want. I realize that, once you've done this, the piece of paper will taunt you, create shame and guilt, and make you feel inadequate. But only if you ignore it.

Here's the thing about goal achievement: writing the goal is simply the primer to get the engine running. It doesn't mean the goal has to be realized tomorrow. Change takes time, so you must keep that goal front of mind as you implement new behaviors and figure out how to break old habits. Put that sticky note on your mirror. Write that goal at the front of your daily journal. Post it on the home screen of your smartphone. Pin it to the wall of your office. Just put it where you can be reminded of it every day. Even if you don't do anything about it.

As days pass without action on that goal you may get irritated, and if that happens long enough, maybe you'll do something about it?

Years ago, I wrote out a list of repairs and chores that I needed to get done around my house and yard before winter.

I was in my early thirties and trying to be a responsible home-owner, so I listed the tasks on a piece of paper and stuck it to my fridge, determined to get that shit done in the next weekend or two. The list included those one-off tasks that get overlooked: fix the broken latch on the gate, get a new padlock for the shed, prune the apple tree, have the lawn mower blades sharpened, clean the garage. Tedious tasks for a single gal with better things to do. And since I had no honey, that "honey-do" list was 100 percent up to me.

The list hit the fridge mid-April. I looked at it all through May. Every time I opened the fridge for breakfast or a snack or dinner, I'd see that list. It hung there through June. I'd go into the freezer for ice cream or ice cubes and that list would taunt me. In July I briefly attempted to prune the apple tree, and my neighbor said I should wait until the growing season was over. So, I put down the shears and picked up the phone and made plans with my friends instead. I procrastinated that list right until the end of summer. And as the air cooled and the leaves started to change, I decided I was sick of looking at that list and it was time to cross off the items.

I completed most of the small tasks in less than an hour. Then I called an arborist to prune the tree and brought the mower blades in for sharpening. That was easy. It took me most of Sunday to clean the garage. Five months of staring at that list and I finally completed it in a day and a half, just so I could get the damn piece of paper off my fridge.

The items on that list were tasks rather than goals, but you get the point. Without the list I would have delayed doing them even longer. Out of sight, out of mind. And although it took me five months, I got that shit done! Imagine if the things on that list had been worthwhile personal or professional goals.

5. Consider key dependencies

One more important aspect of goal setting that most people fail to consider is key dependencies on others. How much will you need to rely on others to achieve your goals? Work-related goals often include key dependencies, especially if you're working on a team objective. Dependencies might include business partners, service providers, or specific co-workers. Professional goals that are yours alone may also rely on key dependencies like a mentor, your boss, a coach, or a trusted colleague. Key dependencies for personal goals may include family members, a hired professional like a personal trainer or web designer, or even someone who might confound your efforts unless you get them onside.

By identifying people who can help you reach your goals, you'll increase your chances of success. Yes, you will have to share your goals with at least one person, but if you communicate what you need from them, the accountability they will provide in return may be a goal-crushing game-changer.

As you craft your goals, list your key dependencies for each, and note what you need to do to get them on board. Then consider these questions for each goal:

Do your key dependencies have goals that complement or conflict with your own?

Are your key dependencies aware of what you need from them to reach your goals?

Are your desired outcomes a priority for them?

If your goal success depends on others, clear communication is crucial, starting from the time you set your goal and continuing until you reach it. Tell people why your goals are important. Make sure all your dependencies know why they are critical to helping you achieve your aims. Enlist people who will champion your efforts, not sabotage them.

We set goals because we ultimately want to achieve them. Implement these five facets of good goals and you will increase the likelihood of great goal achievement.

Time It

In 1955, British historian Cyril Northcote Parkinson wrote an article for the *Economist* that opened with the statement: "It is a commonplace observation that work expands so as to fill the time available for its completion." Essentially, if you have two hours to complete a task, you'll use the entire two hours, even if that task can be completed in less time. And so was born Parkinson's Law.[3]

Use Parkinson's Law to improve how you work. For every task or goal you have in front of you:

- Identify the scope of the task.
- Determine how long it will *realistically* take to complete.
- Create your own time-driven deadline.

If you determine it will take you sixty minutes to complete a short-term task, set a timer for sixty minutes—or, better yet, set a timer for forty-five minutes. Research shows that this simple hack can lead to higher outputs.[4]

During this time, allow no interruptions or distractions. Keep your head down, apply yourself thoroughly to the task, and get it done. If you end up needing more time, that's fine. Do your best to complete the task before the time runs out if it's possible to do so without compromising the quality of your work. And finish early if you can complete the task in less time. Don't drag it out.

For long-term goals, establish a reasonable "achieve by" date, then implement the accountability piece from the SMARTer goals framework I share below. Then get to work.

SMART Goals Are Dumb

It seems any time the topic of goal setting comes up, someone mentions SMART goals. I, for one, am not a fan. In fact, I think SMART goals are pretty dumb.

This standard acronym for goal setting feels uninspiring and safe. Specific and measurable I can grasp, but achievable, realistic, and time-based? Those guidelines don't feel very risky or passion-filled to me. Why set a goal if it doesn't scare and thrill you just a bit?

Good goals are meant to stretch you, to excite you about what's possible, so you chase after them at all costs. You won't reach your goals unless you act, and you're less likely to act on goals that don't invigorate you.

When I was gaining my certification as a professional coach through the Co-Active Training Institute,[5] I was introduced to a more exciting method of goal setting that adds some ART to your SMART. See if you like this method as much as I do.

Thrilling

With traditional SMART goals, you begin by identifying the specific and measurable aspects of your goal, but that's difficult when the goal isn't fully formed. If we begin with the end in mind and work our way up, the process is much clearer.

The T usually asks, "Is your goal timely or time-based?"—meaning, can you achieve it in a reasonable span of time? Time-based goals are good for success because, let's face it, if it takes too long to realize progress, you're more likely to throw in the towel. But to keep things exciting, let's add another T to the mix.

"Thrilling" goals are those that you can't wait to begin. If you establish a goal that really electrifies you (even if it scares you) your chances of success skyrocket. Your goal isn't meant to be something you feel you *should* do. Create a goal that inspires and delights you. Ask yourself, *What possibilities exist for me beyond my goal? What will its completion bring to my life? How will I feel?* Connect to that vision and see what transpires.

I always wanted to run a marathon. As a fitness enthusiast and recreational runner I was thrilled about the idea of one day crossing that finish line, having trained for and run 26.2 miles. I had no idea how it would unfold, what it would take, or when I would do it, but I was fired up by the idea and held on to that vision for several years. I'm certain I would have run the marathon sooner if I knew about this style of goal setting. I'll clarify why in a moment.

Resonant

Setting "realistic" goals might make them easier to achieve, but it likely won't help you grow beyond what you already know. In this SMARTer version of goal setting, we move away from establishing a *realistic* goal toward creating a *resonant* one.

What a great word:

res·o·nant *adj.*
   a. Strong and deep in tone; resounding.

   b. Having a lasting presence or effect; enduring.

   c. Strongly reminiscent; evocative.[6]

If your goals don't resonate with you at a deeper level, they will be harder to stay connected to. Consider these questions: Do you truly want the goal you set? Does it move you toward becoming more of the person you want to be? Does it have a lasting presence in your head and heart as you work on it?

I knew I wanted to run a marathon, but I was rarely clear on when or where, and for some reason I wasn't excited about running my hometown marathon in Calgary, so the goal just sat there. It wasn't until a running friend suggested I travel somewhere interesting to do my marathon that I felt excited. I could combine my love of travel with completing this goal! I mean, who wouldn't love to escape winter and head to Honolulu even if it *is* for a long running race?

Accountable

I've always been a bit irritated by the redundancy of the original A—"achievable"—in the SMART goals model. Don't we set goals *because* we want to achieve them? If you set good goals, you'll achieve them, and the best way to do that is to change this A to "accountable." Having someone hold you accountable to your process is an excellent way to support success.

I know what you're thinking: *The last thing I need is the guilt of failing publicly or having someone scold me if I don't succeed.* But accountability should not be about guilt or nagging; it should be about the right kind of support and focus. Without this step my marathon training would have been a lot tougher. Once I decided to run a destination marathon, I joined a marathon training group with more than thirty other runners who also aimed to run a marathon sometime in November or December of that year. Many of them were training for the Honolulu

Marathon just like me, and our entire eight-month training program was mapped out for us in wonderful detail.

We met Mondays for a short run and strategy lecture, then on Saturdays for a long run, and you can bet that if I missed a run, more than one person would call or email to ask where I was and if I needed a partner for my makeup run. As a group we supported each other, offered guidance, and held each other accountable from start to finish, and everyone in that program finished their chosen marathons.

With the old model of SMART goal setting I could tell myself that training for and running a marathon was absolutely achievable—in fact I did, several times—but it wasn't until I connected accountability to my process that I *achieved* this long-held goal.

Accountability is powerful, as are thrilling and resonant goals. Once you've established these first three elements, the measurable and specific take care of themselves.

Measurable and specific

Make your goal measurable and attach a date to it. This step is essential because it helps you know when you're there. If you want to reduce your credit card debt, you can set a goal to pay off $1,500 by February 15. On that date you'll know whether you succeeded or not. You might also set a goal to lose ten pounds by April 1 or have five website pages built by October 30. All are goals you can measure easily once the specific date arrives. You've either reached the goal or you haven't.

Good goals are also crystal clear in their outcome. What do you want for yourself? "I want to run a marathon someday" doesn't clarify the goal all that much. "I want to run the Honolulu Marathon" gets a little clearer. If I say, "I want to run the Honolulu Marathon next year," visualizing the outcome and getting started is easier. "I will run 26.2 miles on

December 11, 2005, at the Honolulu Marathon" is both measurable and specific.

Do you see how setting SMART (specific, measurable, accountable, resonant, thrilling) goals is far more powerful than setting achievable, realistic, and time-based goals? When we connect our goals to our passions, we add a gripping presence to them and, as if by magic, the goals become achievable.

Engage Your #SuccessEnergy: The Big Little Question

Back in chapter 1 I asked you to start thinking about how you'd answer the big little question: *What do you want?* Now I want you to write down some of those thoughts.

Exploring how to find success with everything that's important to you begins with your goals. Do you know yours? What *do* you want? Do you get up most days excited for what's ahead? What are your goals for your career, finances, relationships, health . . . for your life? When you align what you do and why you do it, you're in a prime position to navigate toward great things. Remember, purpose is a powerful driver of success, and it's one of the key reasons goals matter.

The big little question is not an easy one to answer on the fly. It might even make you uncomfortable at first. Ask it anyway. Before you begin, turn off the censorship button that fills your head with thoughts like, *What I want doesn't matter. Besides, I have no clue! It's impossible, I can't, no time, no energy . . . blah, blah, blah.* Don't listen. If you can dream it, you can do the freakin' work to make it happen.

Go with your gut in answering the big little question that follows, then specify using the seven related questions. Be selfish. Make your responses about you and your vision of success at work, and in the rest of your life. Friends and family may factor into your vision, but try to respond with focused attention on your own needs first. Gift yourself some time right now to start the process. Don't overthink. Point form counts, and you already know why writing it down makes a difference, so pick up a pen and answer away!

What do you want?
What does success look like to you?
What or who is important to you in your daily life?
What's working in your life?
What isn't working?
What or who receives energy from you that they don't deserve?
What needs to change?
What do you want to try?

What do you want? This big little question will help you get to the core of who you are and who you want to be. Keep asking it until the answers appear.

6

MANAGE YOUR MOTIVATION MATRIX

*Thinking is easy, acting is difficult,
and to put one's thoughts into action is
the most difficult thing in the world.*

JOHANN WOLFGANG VON GOETHE

THE FIRST STEP to doing great work is setting great goals. In the formula $S = G \times f(B,D)^E$, once you've figured out what those goals (G) are, the achievement of them becomes a function (f) of the belief (B) you have in yourself regarding those goals, and the discipline (D) within you to do the work. But just because you've set a great goal, that doesn't mean you'll suddenly be motivated to crush it, does it? To drive success with any goal, you must understand the interplay of B and D—your self-belief and self-discipline.

Ideally, we'd approach every goal with shoulders squared, ready to do the work because we want the outcome and we know we're capable. If only it were so simple. Your belief in yourself will often move from high to low, and everywhere in between, depending on the goal you're chasing. You'll also possess varying degrees of discipline toward different goals, so if you can learn to recognize and work through these highs and lows, your likelihood of success will increase.

I've identified four different motivation types based on the levels of belief we have in ourselves and our discipline for a given goal. I call it "The Motivation Matrix."

The Motivation Matrix

Once you've identified a goal, your motivation for it will place you in one of four quadrants on The Motivation Matrix, as you'll see in the following illustration. Based on your goal, you must first determine the level of belief you have in your ability to achieve it. Is it high or low? When you think about the goal, are you mired in self-doubt, or full of confidence and self-efficacy? Next, think hard about how much discipline you possess to do everything necessary to achieve that goal. Assess your current or past behavior: for example, you've attempted this goal before and know that when it gets difficult, you distract yourself. You seem to find other things to do, so you know discipline is low. Also, assess your excitement about the goal. Are you chomping at the bit to get to it, or is your enthusiasm on the low end of the scale?

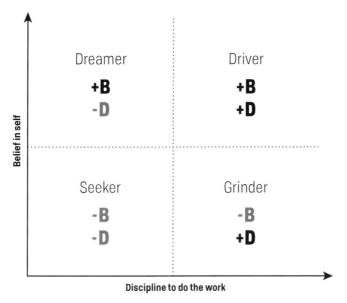

B = Belief in yourself and your goal
D = Discipline to do the work

Whether you're a Dreamer, Driver, Grinder, or Seeker will change for any given goal—personal, professional, short or long term, focused or frivolous. The categories aren't fixed, and you can learn your way toward being the Driver (which is where you want to be) by paying attention to what drives you. Like most people, I've spent time in each quadrant as I've journeyed through my career. This is part of figuring out who we are and who we want to be. Since I clarified what I'm meant to be doing and want to be doing, I've spent more time in the Driver quadrant. Pay attention to what motivates you so you can spend less time seeking, dreaming, and grinding, and more time driving toward that which lights you up. Let's look closer at each of the motivation types.

The Driver

This first motivation type is the gold standard we'd all love to embody for everything we do. The Driver has high belief in themselves and their goal (+B), and high discipline to work toward success (+D). The Driver is good at blocking out distractions, maintaining focus, and staying positive—or at least optimistic—as they work toward success.

We all have the Driver in us. If you have trouble achieving your goals or are easily distracted from the hard work to reach them, you may disagree, but you have it. Possibly the Driver within you is temporarily focused on raising young kids, or driving teenagers around, or fulfilling another obligation. You may believe in your cause and be disciplined enough to see it through, but doing so may feel more like work than like goal chasing. If you're getting the work done, however, and you're not questioning your ability to do it, you're the Driver on those tasks. You may also be the Driver on goals and tasks that might benefit from *less* of your attention. A coaching colleague of mine lamented that her adult son was very good at procrastinating the development of the website for his landscaping business, but he would spend many focused, disciplined hours every evening gaming with his online community.

When does your Driver show up? Which goals or tasks do you embrace with the Driver? Are they worthwhile ways to spend your time? What is it about your positive Driver tasks and goals that make you want to spend time on them?

The Grinder

How often are you faced with tasks that you don't want to work on, but you do the work anyway? The Grinder epitomizes the hard worker, the one who doesn't necessarily love what they do, but they do it because they have to or because they know it will eventually lead to better. The Grinder typically has low belief in themselves and/or what they're doing (-B), coupled with high discipline to do the work (+D) despite that.

On many levels the Grinder is committed to simply doing the work, even if it's hard, and even if it's not something they're passionate about. The Grinder in you might hate doing your taxes, but you grind through it because the alternative—the tax people knocking on your door—isn't appealing. You might hate your job, but you do it because you have a family to care for, and that gives you discipline. You might have low belief in yourself to go after whatever makes your heart sing, but you know you need to pay your bills, so you do the work in front of you, even if it doesn't inspire you. The Grinder will show up when you have a pressing deadline you've avoided until the last minute because it was unappealing, like a boring project, or that university paper, or a difficult conversation. Discipline drives you, even though it feels difficult.

In many ways, the Grinder in you is proof you've got what it takes to do anything you set your mind to. If you've got discipline to work hard despite low belief in yourself or the work in front of you, imagine what you'll be capable of once you find the right work, or learn ways to boost your self-confidence and self-esteem!

When you think about the goals and tasks in front of you, is it the work you struggle with, or your mindset around it? How much does self-esteem hold you back from doing something different? How often do you give yourself credit for staying in the game and doing the work, even when it's hard? If you stopped holding yourself back, what would you do with your life?

The Seeker

There are times when you might feel a little lost or disconnected about certain goals. When you're faced with a task that you're not excited about or don't believe in (-B), and you just don't have the discipline to work at it (-D), you're the Seeker. Seekers might describe themselves as "stuck," especially if low B and D seem to be attached to everything they do. Others might label someone in this space as a "slacker." If you're in this quadrant, you might feel bad because you're not getting things done.

Seekers lack energy for the tasks in front of them. They may be unclear about their goals or not have any. They may be struggling with too many priorities or working on the wrong ones. They may have skills and talents but fail to recognize their strengths. And with low excitement about doing the work, the cycle of apathy can infect other parts of life.

Those stuck in the Seeker quadrant may also need to be more honest with themselves about their work ethic, and some may need to shift their perspective on or attitude about the work they're doing. Which is to say, if you're stuck for a long time, it usually means you need to be doing something different, *or* you're doing the right work but you're lazy, *or* you're doing the right work but you need help and guidance to do it better.

However, if you suffer from anxiety or depression you may fall into the Seeker space during depressive episodes, even if you love what you do. If this is you, get the help you need to navigate the lows, through medication, counseling, or ideally both.

When the Seeker shows up, pay attention to what you're doing and how it makes you feel. What is it about Seeker tasks that cause you to stall? What's getting in the way of your productivity? How can you subtly shift the work to improve it? If you weren't doing this work, what would you be drawn to doing?

The Dreamer

This last motivation type shows up when we have tasks and goals that we know we can do and that we want to achieve (+B), and yet we don't do them (-D). Having high belief and low discipline means you think about your goals more than you act on them.

There are two types of Dreamers. The first lives in a fantasyland full of ideas and big dreams but fails to execute on much of anything. They think more of themselves than they should—they don't get much done and often can't see their shortcomings because they're too busy dreaming up the next big thing. This first type of Dreamer epitomizes "failure to launch," and since I doubt they'd have the sense to pick up a book about how to work better for success at everything, I'll just move on to version two.

The second, more common type of Dreamer is you, me, and anyone else who has a vision of what they want for themselves that just seems to sit there, waiting for them to do something with it: You know you need exercise and believe it will help you feel better, but you don't make the time. You've thought about writing a book for several years, and you know the topic will resonate with many people, but you don't sit down to write. You think about launching a business that interests and excites you, but competing priorities keep it on the back burner. You get the idea. You truly want something for yourself personally or professionally, but you can't find the time, motivation, or energy to tackle it. Here's why that happens.

More often than not in the Dreamer quadrant, tasks compete with all the "have tos" in life. You *have to* take care of your family, you *have to* go to work every day and do what's expected of you, you *have to* deal with emergencies and deadlines (and the fatigue that they bring), you *have to* tackle all the tasks and to-dos that come at you constantly, so many of which you have no control over. All the while, those Dreamer goals patiently wait for you to find the time and energy to get to them. Dreamer tasks also get sidelined by the 21st-and-a-quarter-century distractions that we often choose over doing the work, because we're tired and unmotivated after tackling all those *other* tasks all day long.

What goals are on your "Dreamer list"? How long have those goals been following you? What impacts your discipline to do the work? How would it feel to finally conquer a few of your Dreamer goals?

Get Intentional

Goals are left undone for so many reasons, but mainly because *life*—childcare, emergencies, deadlines, last-minute necessities—obstructs our progress. We want to accomplish our goals, but we don't always prioritize them. So we find ourselves saying, "I'll get to them when..."

A study in the *British Journal of Health Psychology* suggested that wanting the results of a successful goal is often not enough motivation.[1] In this study on motivation and exercise, setting an intention and a plan of action produced far better results than motivation alone. Try this:

- Write down each of your goals.
- Next to each goal, specify your intentions for action.
- Note when, where, and how will you complete the goal.

According to Columbia University professor and success researcher Heidi Grant Halvorson, deciding in advance when and where you will do specific actions to reach your goal may double or triple your chances of success.[2] I like those odds. I mean, why set a juicy goal if you're just going to keep pushing it aside?

Finding Your Drive

The chart that follows provides an at-a-glance look at each motivation type and the barriers and strengths that typify it. If you're procrastinating a task or goal you feel you should complete, establish which barriers seem to be getting in your way, and which motivation type they fall under. It may help you determine why you're stuck and how you can regain momentum.

The Dreamer - D + B =	The Driver + D + B =
Competing priorities	*Clear goals*
Distractions	*Confidence in self*
Fatigue/low energy	*Focus and discipline*
Belief in the dream	*Energy to get it done*
The Seeker - D - B =	**The Grinder** + D - B =
Unclear goals	Unclear goals
Low self-esteem/positive regard	Low self-esteem/positive regard
Distractions/competing priorities	Fatigue/low energy
Fatigue/low energy	*Discipline despite it all*

If your ultimate goal is to become the Driver more often, you can do a few things to help that process. Whether it's your belief in yourself that's low, or your discipline—or both—pay attention to what's going on when you're in those spaces. The Seeker and the Grinder struggle with low belief, which usually boils down to being unclear about a goal, having a flimsy goal, or trying to work at the wrong goal. Spend time reflecting on your goals and do the work to make them as thrilling and resonant as possible, so that you feel excited about them and they ignite action.

Low belief in self may also stem from a lack of unconditional positive regard. Psychologist Carl Rogers defined unconditional positive regard as being accepted, valued, and treated positively regardless of one's behavior.[3] Certainly, our behavior can be influenced by what others think of us, and what we think of ourselves affects how we act. When self-esteem and self-confidence are low, we tend to hold ourselves back from big challenges, even though we may well be capable of doing them. In the next chapter we'll look at how our belief systems are formed, how to troubleshoot negative thinking, and ways to boost self-belief.

When discipline is low, as with the Seeker and the Dreamer, there are often two main culprits: competing priorities and too many distractions. Unfortunately, competing priorities are often necessary tasks, and avoiding them will make your life more difficult. Childcare is a priority, as are family and work obligations. If you have skin in the game of life, no doubt you have quite a few priorities on your to-do list, so don't beat yourself up if you're feeling overwhelmed. Instead, take a closer look at *everything* that's acting on you. Is there anything you can say no to? Are there tasks that you can delegate to others? Can you ask for help so that you can corner a bit of time for the goals you long to work on?

Sometimes the competing priorities are distractions—low-level waste activities that are easier or more fun than the goal-oriented task you procrastinate. You understand what I mean if you've ever said this to yourself: "I really should turn off the TV/put down the iPad/step away from social media and do something more productive!"

Here's an absolute truth that, if you embrace it, will be a discipline game-changer: if you find a way to cut through the noise of 21st-and-a-quarter-century stress and focus in on the work you're truly meant to do, success will be easier won. (Don't worry, help with this will come in chapter 8, when we take a closer look at how to push aside distractions and amp up discipline.)

One barrier common to so many busy people impacts both self-belief and self-discipline: fatigue. The lack of energy you may be feeling is often the result of the poor health you want to change but can't prioritize, from exercise you're not getting to unhealthy eating habits you might lean on when you're busy. It comes from the sleep deprivation that so many people complain about and don't change. It comes from untaken breaks and missed social connections. It comes from bad habits—like smoking, excessive alcohol consumption, or drug use—that impact health, energy, and good judgment.

Once you prioritize health and energy management, though, you'll fuel your push to become the Driver. I cannot wait to share with you the many "small steps" ways you can improve your energy. In chapter 9 I'll do just that!

Engage Your #SuccessEnergy:
Mining Your Motivation Types

At the end of each motivation type description in this chapter, I shared a few questions. You'll find it helpful to write out your answers to each of them to better understand your motivation type tendencies. As you answer the questions, you'll increase awareness of your strengths and blocks, and you'll lay the foundation for the work to come in the chapters that follow.

Here they are again:

The Driver

When does your Driver show up?

Which goals or tasks do you embrace with the Driver? Are they worthwhile ways to spend your time?

What is it about your positive Driver tasks and goals that make you want to spend time on them?

The Grinder

When you think about the goals and tasks in front of you, is it the work you struggle with or your mindset around it?

How much does self-esteem hold you back from doing something different?

How often do you give yourself credit for staying in the game and doing the work, even when it's hard?

If you stopped holding yourself back, what would you do with your life?

The Seeker

What is it about Seeker tasks that cause you to stall?

What is getting in the way of your productivity?

How can you subtly shift the work to improve it?

If you weren't doing this work, what would you be drawn to doing?

The Dreamer

What goals are on your "Dreamer list"?

How long have those goals been following you?

What impacts your discipline to do the work?

How would it feel to finally conquer a few of your Dreamer goals?

AND, FINALLY: What have you learned about yourself through answering the questions above?

7

BUILD BELIEF IN YOURSELF AND YOUR GOALS

---

66 Always remember you are braver
than you believe, stronger than you seem,
and smarter than you think. 99

A.A. MILNE, WINNIE-THE-POOH

Now that you have a better understanding of the interplay between belief (B) and discipline (D) for goal achievement, and perhaps a better sense of the motivation type that drives your behaviors, it's time to take a closer look at belief and how to strengthen it.

Self-belief is having confidence in your own abilities or judgment. When it's high you do great things with more focus and clarity because you spend less time questioning whether you can, whether you should, and even whether you deserve it. You simply accept that you do. With high self-belief comes greater self-esteem. In psychology, self-esteem is used to describe your overall sense of personal value, how much you appreciate and like yourself. If you have low self-esteem, you may not believe that you're capable of success, and this could hold you back. With healthy self-esteem, you are able to navigate life with a positive, assertive attitude and trust you can accomplish your goals, and this can help you achieve.

In The Success-Energy Equation, self-belief (B) is perhaps the most important factor to drive your success. Why? Because it doesn't matter how grand and wonderful your goals are if you don't believe in your ability to crush them. If self-efficacy is low, you'll likely give up on your goals too soon because deep down you don't believe your efforts will make a difference. If you possess high self-efficacy, you're more likely to work harder toward accomplishing a task. When self-esteem and self-efficacy are strong, you possess greater self-confidence in everything you do.

In the previous chapter in our exploration of the motivation types, you learned the two types that possess low B: the Seeker and the Grinder. Unclear goals can cause low self-belief. Fatigue or low energy also influence how you feel about yourself. Often, however, low B stems from low positive self-regard, which will impact your choices and the behaviors that drive your success.

Your Body Hears Everything You Say

What do you say when you talk to yourself? I'm sure you're aware of an inner voice that provides a running monologue in your life, day and night. This inner self-talk—a combination of your conscious thoughts and your unconscious beliefs and biases—is your brain's way of interpreting and processing your daily experiences.

Self-talk can be positive and supportive or negative and defeating. Positive self-talk is the kind of messaging you give yourself throughout the day. Statements like, "I can do whatever I set my mind to" or "I'm calm and confident" or "I got this!" will strengthen your self-assurance and guide you to work through your fears. Positive self-talk has even been linked to the reduction of stress and is good for your mental and physical well-being. So the more you can practice it, the better.[1]

Negative self-talk is that inner dialogue that diminishes you and your ability to make positive changes in your life, and it will weaken self-confidence. Negative self-talk often doesn't reflect our reality and can cause us to act in ways far beneath our capabilities. As thinking, processing humans, unfortunately, our self-talk is more likely to lean toward the negative, with thoughts like, *I'll never be able to do this* or *I'll just fail, so why bother* or *I don't care!*

Negative, in itself, isn't always bad. Negative thinking can heighten our sensitivity to our situation and surroundings. If you're faced with potential danger or adversity, negative thinking will help you assess more clearly. As you walk across a deserted parking lot late at night, your negative self-talk should dominate as you scan your surroundings for potential threats. When you spot a shady-looking individual lurking near your vehicle, that voice inside you should be cautious and wary. *I'm alone and he is bigger than me. What if he's dangerous? I'd better go back to the building and call security. He may be harmless, but he may also be up to no good. Better safe than sorry.*

As you prepare to invest money or hire a contractor or start a business, it's wise to be cautious until you gather enough information to determine whether you're making a sound decision. If those spidey-senses go off and your inner dialogue starts to question or doubt, it's a sign you may need to pay closer attention to what's going on. This logical, accurate version of negative self-talk is grounded in your ability to critically think your way through a situation.

It gets complicated, however, if perception and reality are out of sync, and your negative self-talk overrules reality. You may be a strong and capable person who believes yourself useless after years of being told that you are. You may be a healthy-weight adult but carry feelings of inadequacy stemming from being teased as a "chubby" child. You could be smart and accomplished but continue to play small in your life because you grew up without praise or recognition.

This "inaccurate" version of negative self-talk forms our inner critic—that doubting, cautious, nagging voice that offers up opinions to you about who you are, who you should be, and how you should act. We all have one. It also answers to names like inner gremlin, saboteur, or the devil on your shoulder. No matter what you call it, over time, the negativity of that inner voice will hold you back from realizing your full potential and exact an emotional toll. Are you familiar with what your inner critic says to you?

When I first met Fiona—a past personal training client— she was thirty-two years old and had never been in a gym. She wanted to lose weight and gain energy, but she had very little confidence when it came to exercise, because she'd never really done much of it. During our first few sessions she would show her discomfort by laughing at herself and mocking her lack of ability, even though it was rarely warranted. She would say things like, "I'm such a klutz." "I can't do push-ups, I'm weak." "God, I must be doing this all wrong." And then she'd invariably give up, even though she was capable of more. I would leave those sessions mentally exhausted from the negative energy.

In one of those sessions I suggested she train for a five-kilometer race. She snorted, then blurted out a string of self-deprecating reasons why not, which was when I made her aware of how badly she always talked to herself. She didn't realize the degree to which she hid behind her put-downs. Somehow it brought her comfort, she said. Fiona grew up in a family where she was "the non-athletic one" among her siblings. Her older sister was taller and leaner than she was and played competitive volleyball straight through university. Her younger brother was good at every sport he tried and played hockey and baseball at a high level all through their youth. Fiona, however, was clumsy and uncoordinated, or so they told her every time they did activities together. As a result, she tended to watch from the sidelines when they played, and she began to dislike gym class or physical fitness of any sort. Her inner voice had convinced her she wasn't athletic.

We struck a deal that if I caught her smack-talking herself, she'd have to say something nice to herself, and do ten push-ups, sit-ups, or jumping jacks ... with a smile on her face! And she was going to train for a 5K.

It took self-awareness (and a lot of push-ups), but in the weeks that followed, Fiona spoke more kindly to herself during our workouts, and, not surprisingly, she began to work harder and see more results. She also found out that she liked running, and she was neither incapable nor uncoordinated. She completed her first 5K race only six weeks after she started running, then set goals to run a 10K and a half-marathon that same year, which she also achieved. She became a very strong runner. Once Fiona changed how she talked to herself, she began to experience greater success with her goals and was more content with her life in general.

The moral of the story: Pay attention, because your body hears everything you say. Negative self-talk is linked to higher levels of stress and lower self-esteem.[2] Low self-esteem causes you to carry yourself with less poise and confidence, and you'll often go through the day feeling fatigued, anxious, or even depressed. Fatigue, anxiety, and depression can lessen your ability to see opportunities around you, and if you do see them, you may be less inclined to capitalize on them. Negative self-talk also influences how you speak with others, often fostering self-deprecating messaging about yourself and your abilities.

This behavior can strain relationships and position you in such a way that others will fail to recognize your true nature and talents. You might be the best person for the promotion, but you get overlooked because you downplay your worth in front of your boss. You may have a kind heart and good intentions, but your friends tire of your constant complaining and negativity, so they avoid you.

Your body hears everything you say, your subconscious brain believes what it hears most often, and the strongest message always wins. So it's worthwhile to learn how to improve your self-talk.

Self-Esteem and
21st-and-a-Quarter-Century Stress

Check in with how the digital noise of 21st-and-a-quarter-century stress plays on your belief in yourself. There are a few significant influences:

Social media

We feel pressure to curate interesting, like-worthy social channels—to look good, to appear successful, and to have an interesting life—and we can waste a lot of time and emotional energy doing so.

The more time we spend scrolling our social channels, the more likely we are to get caught up in energy-draining social comparison. Our stress increases and our self-worth declines.

We see what we post as an extension of who we are. Every update, picture, and activity we share makes us fodder for marketers who try to sell us products we didn't know we needed for problems we didn't know we had.

We derive a false sense of belonging from social media. We give too much time and energy to our hundreds or thousands of online pseudo-friends and neglect our face-to-face friends.

Real life and all the wonderful people and experiences in it are constantly interrupted by the need to share it all on our social media channels. We're not fully present to the moment because we stop to take the interesting photo, edit it perfectly, come up with a clever comment, and make sure we include all the right hashtags before posting.

Daily news

We get negative and stressful news from across the globe at all hours of the day, moments after it happens, so we never take a mental break from the chaos.

Much of the news is increasingly visual and shocking because of the inclusion of bystander-captured video and audio clips, and can lead to sleep problems, anxiety, and even PTSD-like symptoms.[3]

We want to stay informed, but processing fact versus sensationalism is increasingly difficult, leading to stress and uncertainty.

Our ingrained negativity bias means we're wired to pay attention to information that scares or unsettles us, and there's a lot more of that these days, so our stress response is taxed.

Information overload

The internet can answer any question we have about our goals and ideas. Just google it! Unfortunately, it can also uncover a lot of information we don't need, like whether our idea has been done before, where, and by how many others. Information overload and social comparison can lead to apathy and may impact progress and self-confidence.

It's hard to stay on top of it all—news, social channels, latest technologies, learning opportunities, must-read books, must-watch programs—and *not* feel stressed, overwhelmed, or inadequate.

WHICH OF the above can you relate to? Are you starting to feel convinced that simplifying your digital life might boost your energy? Pay attention to how media of all sorts impacts your self-esteem and self-confidence. If feelings of stress, overwhelm, or worthlessness creep in while you're online, get off. Take a break for a few hours or more, reduce your information intake for a few days, decide what you can live without. Your self-esteem will thank you.

Think Like Forrest

If you're familiar with the 1994 movie *Forrest Gump*, starring Tom Hanks, you'll remember that Forrest achieved moments of greatness throughout his life—some would say far beyond what might be expected of him, and despite being branded as unintelligent at a young age.

Today Forrest might be called autistic,[4] and our first impression of someone like him might be that life would be harder for him, and he might not accomplish much. Yet, in the movie, Forrest becomes a college football star, is hailed as a war hero after returning from Vietnam, makes worldwide news during a 15,000-mile run through the U.S., and builds a successful shrimping company. He even invests in "some kind of fruit company," which turns out to be Apple Computer. Sure, Forrest Gump is a fictional character, but the question of *how* he comes to such success against the odds operates as a good reminder of what can happen when we improve the way we talk to ourselves. Slow-witted Forrest Gump never thinks of himself as disadvantaged. No part of his brain censors his thoughts or tells him he isn't smart enough, or strong enough, or that no one will take him seriously. As a result, he can dream it and then do it. His supportive mother, played by Sally Field, also has a hand in his success because she never tells him he can't. He believes he can, so he does, and experiences success beyond *our* wildest dreams. Yet we're all capable of greatness beyond our wildest dreams. And it starts with how we talk to ourselves.

Unfortunately, according to behavioral psychologists, as much as 77 percent of self-talk is negative, or works against you, and it takes as many as twenty positive statements about yourself or your situation to counteract even one negative personal statement.[5] Researchers have learned that the human brain operates much like a personal computer. Once information is imprinted on the hard drive, the only way to change it is to erase or replace the information—otherwise, the computer will repeat what you preprogrammed into it. The subconscious mind works in a similar fashion. Information is fed into it through our senses, our thoughts, our impressions, and what we hear from ourselves and others. *I'm such a loser! I can't do this. It's going to be another crappy day.* With messaging like that, it most certainly will be, because we don't like to be wrong, even if being wrong means suffering.

If you haven't learned how to manage it, that inner critic will make you excessively alert to your limitations and hold you back from bigger things. It wants to keep you inside your comfort zone, safe and "close to home" like when you were a kid. Like a concerned, well-intentioned caregiver, it tries to protect you from getting hurt and standing out too much. In fact, that inner messaging may have been imprinted when you were young, with the words of your parents, siblings, or other guardians. The messages may have been relevant when you were little, but as an adult, they may be holding you back.

Here's another important bit of news about your inner critic: it doesn't like change. So, as you step outside that comfort zone toward your goals and dreams, its voice gets louder and attempts to draw you back in: *Not so fast, let's think about this some more. Are you sure you want to risk embarrassment or failure? The work will be hard. I'm not sure you're up for it. Who will take you seriously, anyway?*

Just like an overly protective parent, that inner critic stops you from growing and exploring, from becoming who you're truly meant to be. But as a full-grown, free-thinking adult, you don't have to listen to it. With awareness, you can shut off those messages. With practice, you can shift toward the positive. This is oh so worth it as you drive the road to success, because everything good happens *outside* your comfort zone.

Breaking Out of Your Comfort Zone

Let's talk about this intriguing comfort zone. Its name suggests that it's a good place to hang out, like a cozy lounge full of comfy chairs, but don't be deceived. Typically, the only thing comfortable about your comfort zone is the familiarity you have with it. The dictionary defines the comfort zone as "a place or situation where one feels at ease or secure"[6] or "a settled method of working that requires little effort and yields only barely acceptable results."[7] While it's OK to want ease and a sense of security in your surroundings, if you spend too much time in that unchallenging space, you'll limit your growth. Plus, it will be far easier to settle into "barely acceptable results." Which are unacceptable.

We each design our comfort zone based on our beliefs, experiences, and capacity, and our inner critic has a hand in the design as well. Bad things may be happening in your life right now, but you're familiar with them, and change is hard, so *better the devil you know.*

You may hate your job, but your inner critic advises that you know the job well, it has good benefits, and you don't really want the hassle or stress of looking for more exciting work, so you stay in that uncomfortable comfort zone. You may be in a loveless relationship, but your inner critic reminds you that you know how to manage it and you can't imagine being single again at this age, so you stay stuck. You think about going back to school or taking the promotion, but it would mean more work, and you're not sure you have what it takes, so you tell yourself things are fine as they are. Inner critic. You wonder what it would be like to learn guitar, or join a gym, or take a dance class, but you don't want to risk looking stupid, so you don't do it. The examples are endless, but they have one thing in common: they hold you back from experiencing a more fulfilling, more successful life.

If your inner critic is loud and unruly, the walls of your comfort zone will feel thicker, and it will be harder to step outside it. You'll look beyond its walls toward those things you dream of for yourself, and the gap between where you are now and where you want to be will feel big and overwhelming. As you reach outside that comfort zone your inner critic will get even louder, and to silence the noise you'll be inclined to step back into it, curl up in your La-Z-Boy, and embrace status quo.

If you don't learn how to manage your inner critic, then every time you stretch outside that comfort zone toward better, every time you get close to achieving a goal, that voice will pipe up with fear, self-doubt, or anxiety. It will attempt to draw you back toward the comfort zone, away from the change it so detests, and away from the growth you so deserve. If you learn to manage your inner critic, the voices will still rumble every now and then, but they won't be as loud, and you will know how to shut them down. Moving away from your comfort zone will be easier. When you stretch toward the worthwhile and interesting, instead of being met with overwhelm you'll feel the pull of opportunity. The more often you venture into that space, the more confident you will become in your ability to do what you've always dreamed of.

What If Your Inner Critic Is Wrong?

In the #SuccessEnergy segment at the end of this chapter, I share an exercise that will help you identify your inner critic and get to know it better so that, if you haven't already, you can start to manage it. It's a powerful exercise because it will help you better recognize when your inner dialogue is something you should listen to or something you should question. It will also help you realize just how wrong the inner critic can be sometimes.

When I went through the exercise during my coach training many years ago, it made me angry... at myself. For so many years I had let my inner critic tell me who I was, who I should be, and how I should act. Which made me question everything I did. I spent most of my thirties feeling like I wasn't good enough. I was thirty when I finished grad school with a master's in kinesiology, and I had a good idea of how I wanted my life to unfold now that school was finally done: build a great career as a speaker, educator, and coach; meet the man of my dreams; travel; have experiences; get married; buy a house; get a dog; live a glorious life!

I could envision where I wanted to go in my life, but I wasn't progressing as I wanted. More accurately, my self-belief held me back from getting results sooner. I definitely worked hard, but despite all my effort, I was mired in self-doubt and self-imposed setbacks. I felt like I was stuck on a big treadmill, sweating it out and not getting anywhere as friend after friend whizzed by, arm in arm with their perfect mate, achieving their goals, living their amazing lives. I was building a speaking business focused on helping other people have more life balance, better health, and more happiness, yet I had none of it in my own life. I was an unmotivated motivational speaker.

I called myself a health expert, but I skipped my own workouts, ate poorly, and didn't get enough sleep. I was a tired, out-of-shape personal trainer and that wasn't good for my business or my health. I lived in a place I couldn't afford with roommates I didn't like, working four part-time jobs and living paycheck to paycheck. Plus, I was so focused on my own drama that I made no time for my friends. When I did, I was self-centered, superficial, and needy, which they eventually tired of. Right around that time, I got sideswiped by a bad case of "I suck" when three of my closest friends unfriended me... and that was before Facebook, so it was literally in my face.

All this, *plus* chasing down my future Prince Charming at every turn. I met some nice men, but I carried a feeling of not being good enough into every relationship, which manifested as clingy co-dependency. Not surprisingly, despite being intelligent, attractive, fun-loving, outdoorsy, athletic, and kind, I struggled to maintain those relationships. Despite being a good conversationalist and a great cook, I struggled. Even once I started to earn a steady income and managed to buy my own house and car, I f#%*ing struggled. For almost ten years.

When I look back on that time of my life, I recall a sense of urgency to do everything "right"—to build the career, to establish myself with a home and relationship, to make something of myself as quickly as I could. I wanted to do a good job at something, anything. I wanted to be appreciated, and I cared too much about what others thought of me. I was unhappy, but I covered it up well.

During all those years of struggle, most of my friends thought I had it all together. Despite that inner turmoil (or perhaps *because* of it), by the end of my thirties I had slowly but surely "made shit happen" in my life. I was well educated, I was in management at the fitness club, and my speaking business was gaining momentum. To others, my life looked just great, but to me, something was missing. My outward self was plucky and confident, but my inward self… not so much. A friend I'd confided in at the time called me a beautiful disaster: driven, smart, and put-together on the outside, miserable and unworthy on the inside.

And then one of my long-time personal training clients did something unexpected that opened my eyes to the truth.

Donna and I met a couple of times each week for morning training sessions and had been doing so for more than two years. She was cheerful, easygoing, and we always had good conversations and lots of laughs during our sessions. When I met her on this particular day, she was in her work clothes.

So, I said, "What's up?" She seemed a bit tentative and asked me to sit down on the bench next to her.

She said, "You're a good trainer, and I'm grateful for all you've done for me. The thing is, I come to our sessions to get energized..."

My stomach clenched. *This doesn't sound good. What is she about to tell me?*

"But right now," she said, "you are carrying the weight of the world on your shoulders and I can feel it."

I felt stunned, and a bit confused. *Weight of the world? How can she even see that?*

"You're unhappy," she continued. "I love you, but right now I need to work with a different personal trainer. And you should work with my therapist."

Ouch! *She's firing me!*

A mix of anger, disbelief, and embarrassment surged through me, followed by a little relief. Because she was right. I was unhappy. And if I wasn't fooling her, I probably wasn't fooling too many other people.

So, then and there, I decided it was time to reevaluate my life. I started to see a counselor, which opened a Pandora's box of low self-worth and self-esteem that I'd probably started cultivating in my teenage years. Through my counselor I learned about co-dependency and people-pleasing, and how it manifested itself in my life. I craved approval and got it by working hard and getting results, but it was so I could prove to myself and others that I was worthy. And it was also to silence that damn inner critic.

With that awareness, I picked up a big ol' mirror and took a good hard look at the part I played in the story of my life. I'd been listening to that inner voice for too long, and she had led me off course. Once I realized that I was stuck in a holding pattern in my life, the first thing I did was stop dating. How could

I possibly know what I needed for myself if I was always giving my energy to other people and their needs? I got to know myself better by asking myself the big little question: *What do you want, Michelle?*

I wish I could tell you that I knew the answers right away. Those early days of self-reflection were challenging because not only did I have no clear idea of what was important to me, but also, somewhere deep down, I wondered if I even deserved to have it—whatever *it* was. But I kept asking.

As I pondered the question daily, I first noticed what I *didn't* want, with work, relationships, activities, opportunities, even with what I ate. I started to pay attention, and in the process I got to know myself better. I learned to like myself, and I grew to understand that my health, happiness, and success is, was, and will always be 100 percent up to me. I strengthened neglected friendships, reconnected with past passions (travel, sea kayaking, road trips with girlfriends, *hello*), tried new things (discovering I'm a mountain biker and a dog person through and through), and figured out what is truly important to *me* in my work and my life. I reclaimed my health by eating better, drinking less alcohol, and amping up my fitness regimen. I strengthened my focus on building my speaking business by saying no to side jobs that didn't fuel that goal or fulfill me. I determined that I'm a coach and not a personal trainer, even though I'm very qualified to do both.

By asking myself the big little question daily, I found my answers and was finally able to accept that the authentic version of me—as quirky, in-your-face, and imperfect as I am—is better than any version I made up to please other people.

I share my inner critic story because I want you to know that I've been there, and I can assure you that with the right tools and a bit of practice it's possible to silence that inner critic and realize your true path in life.

Your Brain on Negativity

Why do most of us spend more time dwelling on poor feedback, our mistakes, or someone's unkind words than we do on the positive? Well, negative events have a far greater effect on our gray matter than positive ones. Psychologists refer to this as the negativity bias. Leading brain researcher Rick Hanson says the brain is like Velcro for negative experiences, but like Teflon for positive ones.[8]

Evolutionarily, our negativity bias helped our species survive. Our early ancestors had to make critical decisions several times a day: approach a reward or avoid a risk. Our brains are wired for caution—to zero in on bad news, to downplay good news, and to walk around with a bit of anxiety running through us so that we stay alert. That anxiety originates in the amygdala, which acts as the alarm center of our brain and is responsible for the fight-or-flight stress response to threats. Once it fires up, negative events "go Velcro." As a result, we tend to over-learn from negative experiences and use them as evidence to cement the stories we tell ourselves that hurt our relationships, limit our ambitions, justify our excuses, and suck the happiness from our lives.

To offset this natural human tendency in yourself, try these strategies:

- Hold positive messages in awareness for twelve to twenty seconds, to transfer them from short-term to long-term memory.
- Prioritize positive messaging over your inner critic's negative voice.
- Be kinder and gentler with yourself.
- Practice the 4 Rs for shifting beliefs (see below).

The 4 Rs for Shifting Beliefs

Our thoughts are powerful and they're not always right. If your inner critic is feeding you too much inaccurate information—about what you deserve, what you're capable of, or what other people think—there is a simple process that can help you manage that negative voice. It's called the 4 Rs for shifting belief, and it looks like this:

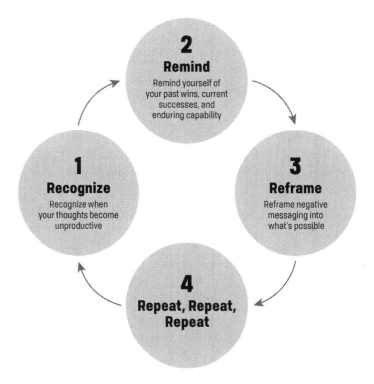

Recognize

Recognize when your thoughts become unproductive. When you hear your inner dialogue shift toward negativity or self-defeating messaging, stop yourself. Notice without judgment what circumstance triggered your inner critic. Simply use your awareness as a learning moment. As you pay attention to how you talk to yourself, you'll realize how often negative thinking happens and why, and you'll be more likely to catch yourself before your thinking goes off the rails.

Remind

Remind yourself of your past wins, current successes, and enduring capability. When negativity takes over, you might overlook the positive stuff going on in your life, as if it has all been covered over with gray paint. But it's there, and usually in greater abundance than you even know—you just have to look harder to see it.

Think about all of your *past wins*. Look back on the events where you experienced success through hard work, got through a trying situation, or completed something you thought would be impossible: work triumphs, getting through school, running that race, recovering from a divorce, the kids you raised into great adults, the health scare you battled back from. Past wins are reminders that if you did it before, you've got the capacity to do it again.

Think about your *current successes*. Today, right now, what are you proud of in relation to the work you do? Who are you grateful to have in your circle? In what ways are your health, finances, career, and relationships working well? Acknowledge the big, small, and everything-in-between successes, because they're all happening in part because of you.

Here are three ways to really imprint those successes in your mind:

Be grateful

Start your day by writing down three things you're grateful for. A daily gratitude practice improves physical health. Grateful people experience fewer aches and pains, are more likely to report feeling healthy, and are more likely to exercise and get regular checkups from their doctor, which improves longevity. A daily gratitude practice also improves psychological health. Leading gratitude researcher Robert Emmons conducted several studies on the link between gratitude and well-being. His research confirms that gratitude effectively increases happiness and decreases depression. Practicing gratitude increases your empathy toward others and reduces aggression, even when others have been less kind to you. Gratitude also helps you sleep better. Research has shown that if you take time *before* bed to write down what you're grateful for, you may sleep better and longer. It improves our self-esteem too, reducing social comparisons—which, in this hyper-connected online world, is a powerful thing.[9]

Write your "amazing list"

I use this exercise with my coaching clients to help them recognize their own greatness. Write a list of fifteen things about yourself that you think are amazing. Most of my clients meet this "amazing list" activity with discomfort and resistance. *I can't come up with that many things. That will be too hard. Do I have to?*

This is a challenging exercise for many because we don't often spend time singing our own praises. When we're young we're told not to brag. We're taught that humility is a virtue. As adults we may choose to downplay our strengths or dismiss them as ordinary, for fear of judgment or to avoid standing out. We dilute our amazingness, and don't give ourselves credit for being special in any way.

But you are, so try the exercise. Take fifteen minutes to write down fifteen amazing things about you. Assume that no one else will see the list and be really honest about what you like about yourself, what you're most proud of, what you're great at. These things make you amazing! Be unlimited about what you deem as amazing! I recently found my own amazing list from 2011. I had twenty-three things on that list, including "I make people laugh and feel good about themselves. I am one hell of a snowboarder. I am a good 'doggie momma' to Lilly. I am full of good ideas that I actually implement. I walk my talk in life. I grow really great tomatoes."

If you want an additional layer of confirmation of your amazingness, try this fun extension. After you've created your own list—and without showing that list to anyone—ask one or two trusted friends, your spouse, or your kids what *they* think is amazing about you. Trust me, it'll be worth it. If you need a prompt, you can tell them you're reading this book and the crazy author suggests you do this. The responses will surprise you, warm your heart, and even make you cry (happy tears). The people who love us see things in us that we don't always see or acknowledge as special, so ask them and take in all the great responses. You're amazing.

Create an "awesome jar"

Several years ago, I sent out a year-end email to my coaching clients asking them, among other things, what they were most proud of that year, and which accomplishments they were celebrating. A week later, when I was on a call with one of them, she said to me that the exercise was challenging for her because while she'd experienced success that year it was through a series of small wins, and she couldn't remember many of them. So, she created an "awesome jar."

She found a big jar, labeled it, and placed it on her desk at work. When something happened that made her proud, she'd write the details on a small piece of paper with the date and stick it in the jar. Whenever she had a personal or professional success—even a small one—she did this. Over the course of the year she recorded dozens of awesome moments as reminders of the success she created in her life.

Anytime she needed a boost she'd stick her hand in the jar and grab a few to read. Then one day a co-worker gave her a nice piece of feedback about her work, and she decided to add another element to her awesome jar. If she received a compliment or positive feedback from someone, she'd ask them to write it on a different color of paper and add it to the jar. Or she'd do it herself. My client created a reminder system for positive feedback about herself that was simple, fun, and effective. Try this for yourself.

AT THE core of a strong belief in self is having a clear understanding of what's great about you, and the greatness you bring to all you do. These are just three ways to remind yourself of your past wins, current success, and enduring capability, and while they may seem a bit simplistic, it is that simplicity that in fact makes them so powerful. You can do them quickly, you can do them often, and you can begin to own your awesome in a bigger way.

Reframe

The third step for shifting beliefs is to reframe negative messaging into what's possible. So often when your inner critic pipes up, it's with self-deprecation and defeatist thinking. Let's say you want to go back to school part-time to further your education, but you're dismayed because the tuition is higher than you hoped, the commute to night classes is lengthy, and the course load might make it difficult to simultaneously work full time. You really want this, yet in frustration you say to yourself, *It can't be done!* Your brain accepts that message, determines that no more processing of this problem is necessary, and shuts off any further conscious or subconscious exploration associated with it.

Rather than shut the door on possibility, reframe to what *is* possible. When you allow yourself to be curious, to brainstorm ways around your barriers, you're more likely to stick with a problem long enough to reach a favorable outcome. A simple way to do this is with "how might I" questions that help you think openly and creatively.[10] "How might I get the extra money for tuition? How might I capitalize on the long commute? How might I balance full-time work and part-time school? How might I get the support I need?" As soon as you reframe your negative thinking into a problem-solving question, your brain switches on and begins to seek out answers to your questions. As you pose a question, give yourself permission to brainstorm every and any possibility. Stay open-minded and be creative:

How might I get the extra money for tuition?
Ask parents
Ask boss for work sponsorship
Start a GoFundMe campaign
Seek out scholarships and bursaries
Find another part-time job
Throw a garage sale
Reduce spending
Get a roommate

Brenda, an attendee at one of my presentations, shared with me that she faced this very problem. She was a full-time administrative assistant at the municipal offices in her hometown, and she wanted to go back to school to become a special education assistant. She didn't have the money, she couldn't wrap her head around the commute, and she wondered how she'd find the time to work *and* study.

By using the "how might I" method, she became more creative and courageous with her problem solving. She sought out local bursaries for mature students and found two that would grant part of her tuition. Her parents offered to help with some of her school expenses as well. She spoke with her boss, who agreed to a flexible schedule that would allow her to telecommute one day each week and take every other Friday off. She would commute to class by bus to save money, and use that time to read and study, and when her school workload increased, she'd work reduced hours at her job or use some of her holiday time for studying and exam prep. "How might I" allowed Brenda to reframe the seemingly impossible goal of going back to school into an exciting reality she was confident she could achieve.

Whenever you're faced with a challenge you view as insurmountable, ask yourself "how might I" questions and recognize the power of possibility.

Repeat ... repeat ... repeat

Our belief systems and the negative messages we send ourselves have been hardwired over many years, so it takes time to erase them and replace them with kinder, more supportive inner dialogue. The Recognize and Reframe strategies I've shared are effective ways to facilitate the shift from negative self-talk to positive. Repetition is vital, because initially those attempts at positive self-talk will feel uncomfortable and even phony. But persevere.

Developing a couple of positivity mantras to repeat throughout the day can help. The "power of positive thinking" is an age-old practice that can seem hokey, especially if you don't feel particularly positive about yourself or some aspect of your life, but when in doubt, *fake it until you make it.* Design your positivity mantras to lead you toward a more optimistic and encouraging inner voice.

Affirmations are powerful. Thoughts, spoken words, and written statements are acts of creation. When writing your

positivity mantra, it's important that your words be in align-
ment with your desires. Develop positivity mantras that
resonate with you and are repeatable when negativity creeps
in and that inner voice reverts to its derisive ways.

Here are some examples to get you started:

"I am good enough. Actually, I'm great!"
"I am healthy in all areas of my life."
"I am funny, loveable, and smart."
"I am full of great ideas and the ability to make them happen."
"I am strong enough to do anything I set my mind to."
"Yes, I can!"

Have some fun with it and don't be afraid to get a bit cheeky
with your mantras. I have three positivity mantras that I repeat
to myself regularly. The first I got from a pair of socks I own:
"Kick this day in its sunshiny ass!" It energizes me and makes
me laugh, so I put it on my bathroom mirror where I can see
it at the start of every day. The other two—"I ROCK!" and
"I GOT THIS!"—I keep posted on my office wall to remind
me that even when I may not feel like a grounded, strong
motivational speaker and coach, I'm pretty awesome and
super-capable. Because I am. We all are. This includes you, so
make sure your positivity mantras reflect that, then repeat . . .
repeat . . . repeat until you believe what you're saying to yourself.

Engage Your #SuccessEnergy: I.D. Your Inner Critic

To stop feeding your inner critic, you must first identify it. Give
it a name and even an avatar, such as the grumpy old man, the
mean schoolmarm, the hyena. This process will help you isolate
your inner critic and treat it as a separate entity, like another
individual whom you can choose to listen to or not. Consider
the following, and record your answers to the questions:

Notice when your inner critic shows up.

What triggers it?

What are you doing or attempting when it comes around?

Pay attention to what it says to you.

What are its favorite sayings or stories? Notice the stories and opinions it constantly shares with you to influence you or your decisions.

Does your inner critic's voice sound familiar? Describe how it sounds and what it looks like. Does it have a name?

Connect its words to your actions.

How does your inner critic attempt to sabotage your actions? Your inner critic delights in giving you bad advice: "Don't speak up. No one cares what you have to say." "Don't ask for the promotion. You'll be rejected." "Forget about relationships. You're not all that loveable." "Skip the gym. Who cares about your health?" "Stop working so hard on that website. Your business dream is a stupid one." Listen for it so you can notice how it influences your behavior.

Change your behavior.

How might you do things differently? Once you know how your inner critic influences your behavior, you can consciously choose to do something different, aligned with positive self-belief. This might feel uncomfortable at first, but it can also feel empowering. Do your best to ignore your inner critic and take a small step toward whatever it's trying to talk you out of. This will take practice and a bit of self-compassion. But the more you do it, the easier it will become to listen to your true heart and act in accordance with it.

PART III

REALLY GET SH!T DONE

8

UNLEASH DISCIPLINE

---

66 Without effort, your skill is nothing more than what you could have done but didn't. 99

ANGELA DUCKWORTH

O NE OF MY favorite books is a short, no-holds-barred read called *Do the Work* by Steven Pressfield. It gets to the core of why, on our path to success, we often get stuck, even when we're working toward something we really want. Pressfield's book is a great reminder that just because we want something—success, fame, health, wealth—and even when we're capable of doing what it takes, we may not always be filled with the motivation and discipline to do it.

He says it like this: "Our enemy is not lack of preparation; it's not the difficulty of the project, or the state of the marketplace, or the emptiness of our bank account. The enemy is resistance. The enemy is our chattering brain, which, if we give it so much as a nanosecond, will start producing excuses, alibis, transparent self-justifications, and a million reasons why we can't/shouldn't/won't do what we know we need to do."[1]

Frustrating, really. So many of us are capable of so much more than we even know, if we could just get out of our own way and do the work. Present company included.

For many years, lack of that do-the-work discipline was the anchor that held me down as I developed my speaking business. When I first started out, I did what was necessary to garner a somewhat regular paycheck: I built a website, reached out to clients, developed my presentations, and improved my skills. I was hungry. Alberta, Canada, the oil province I live in, was experiencing a boom, and I earned a piece of it presenting my life-balance and stress-management topics to busy, stretched professionals. Business was steady and inside of three years I established myself as a full-time professional speaker. I was doing all right, but I wasn't doing great. I dabbled in sales outreach, I didn't have a real business plan, and most of the time I relied on luck, fate, and chance to help me grow my business. They're not very good business partners.

When the 2008 economic downturn hit, I remember cockily telling a colleague, "If there's a recession, I'm choosing not to take part." That's a pretty bold statement from someone who didn't have a solid plan. Turns out, business is often better when the economy is great—even when you don't have a plan. In the fall of 2009, more than 40 percent of my business vaporized. The phone stopped ringing, and the emails stopped coming. I'd reach out to clients and get messages like "all non-essential spending has been frozen" or "our budgets have been cut," or "all staff training has been put on hold … we're sorry."

When business was good, I coasted along and collected the checks; the work found me. When business was good, I was less inclined to do the sales calls I dreaded. My website needed improvements, but I told myself, *It's good enough.* I thought about writing a book, but I was too busy making money to find the time. When business was good, I didn't think about secondary income streams, because I thought I didn't need it. When business was good, there were always things I could do to make it great, but I would procrastinate, prioritize other tasks, or settle for "good enough" with whatever I was working on, because work was steady. But that recession was another animal entirely.

In fairly short order I was having trouble paying my bills. I was single at the time, so there was no second income to lean on, and since the last thing I wanted was to admit defeat and go back to my old job, I got angry with myself for letting things come to that point. Then, I squared my shoulders and did what I should have done at the start. I finally began treating my business like a business. I finally began doing the necessary work to have a strong, sustainable operation.

In the nearly eighteen months that my business struggled, I took sales training and created a workable sales strategy. And I made those damn calls, even when I didn't want to. I finally wrote my first book, *Energy Now! Small Steps to an Energetic Life*, often in the evenings, even when I didn't want to, so I'd be free during the day to go to events and connect with clients. The book provided new speaking opportunities to a wider audience and helped me hone my message. I finally took coaching courses and got certified as a professional coach, which not only provided a secondary income stream but also made me a better speaker. Why? Because the challenges of my coaching clients reflect what my audiences also need help with. My clients keep me current.

For several months, as I rebuilt my business, I coached clients and worked my sales plan, even when I didn't want to. I faced endless rejections from would-be clients until I learned how to effectively sell. I wrote a business plan, six years after I'd launched my business. Whenever I was dragged down by self-doubt, laziness, or the desire to do something else, I'd say to myself, *Just do the freakin' work, Cederberg. DTFW!* I kept doing the freakin' work until business improved. And when it did, I didn't sit back and collect the checks, I kept DTFW front of mind and stayed the course. In fact, I hung a sign on my office wall as a daily reminder that success requires effort. Period.

So, if you take nothing else from this chapter, at least take this: The success you crave has little to do with education, upbringing, or natural ability. It's not about who you know, or how much support you get from family or friends. It's about discipline.

Success comes down to discipline, and discipline means setting your sights on the goal and, even when you don't feel like it, doing what it takes because you know it will bring results. It's about how you work—and when you learn how to work better at the things that matter, it's a game-changer.

Recall that in The Success-Energy Equation—$S = G \times f(B,D)^E$—discipline (D) is foundational for success at anything. If you want success, you need the discipline to work at what will help you get it. Simple, not easy.

If you ask people what holds them back from higher levels of success, they'll usually say they lack focus or direction. They may admit they lack tenacity, or they've become complacent. They might also struggle with poor time management, too many distractions, or too many competing priorities. All these barriers come down to a lack of discipline. When you think about the goals you haven't yet achieved, you might say, *Well, obviously I lack discipline*. That's not entirely true, though. It may be true that you have no discipline for the goal you procrastinate, but it's not true to say you have no discipline at all. More accurate might be to say that your discipline is misdirected.

In the busyness of life, as you navigate daily demands, as you do your job and raise your kids, you channel a great deal of discipline every day. But you may lack discipline for a specific goal. It may also be fair to say that you need to prioritize differently. Everyone has discipline for something, even if that's binge-watching Netflix, or spending all afternoon surfing the internet.

Discipline and 21st-and-a-Quarter-Century Stress

In chapter 6, I shared The Motivation Matrix and the four motivation types. If you recall, Dreamers have high belief in themselves and their goals (+B) but low discipline (-D). Seekers have both low belief (-B) and low discipline (-D). For these motivation types, D may be low because they struggle with too many competing priorities, or they've allowed distractions to sideline their efforts, or, in the case of Seekers, they may be unclear about their goals. Discipline also weakens when fatigue or low energy are constant, which we'll talk more about in the next chapter.

These days, discipline is most often tested by the many competing priorities and daily distractions of 21st-and-a-quarter-century stress. If you don't like the work you're doing, or you're bored, or you need a break, it's near impossible to ignore the lure of games, apps, social media, and non-stop news that calls to you from your smartphone. As you reach for it, the calming effects of dopamine set in, and once you engage, you'll no doubt spend more time scrolling and tapping than you'd like. It's all so enticing . . .

Discipline, however, requires effort and focus. It demands that you block out distractions, address fatigue, prioritize effectively, and do what you commit to, even when you don't want to. Discipline is strengthened when you get clear about what you want. That's why the first two variables of The Success-Energy Equation are so important: when you take the time to formulate thrilling, resonant goals (G), and strengthen your self-belief (B) about achieving those goals, the excitement and confidence that result will increase your desire to do the work. Then, all you'll need to do is find the time and energy, right? Great in theory, I know.

Every day, life happens to you, and you spend most of your time dealing with it. In the busyness, it's tempting to defer work on even the juiciest goals so that you can put out other fires. You look wistfully toward those goals and say to yourself, with the best of intentions, *I'll get to it when I'm not so busy* or *I'll get to it when I'm not so darn tired.* Then, well-intentioned though you may be, life just keeps pulling you toward other, more pressing matters. Or the sofa sucks you in because it's been another long, tiring day. Or you choose to zone out with low-priority tasks because you don't have the bandwidth to dig into your goals.

You still have to do the work to remedy the situation, and with a little awareness you can. But it does require a closer look at how you spend your time.

Pause and Plan

When you're stressed, your sympathetic nervous system triggers the release of adrenalin and cortisol, which causes increased heart rate, blood pressure, and breathing rate. Your pupils dilate, blood rushes from your gut to the working muscles, and blood-sugar levels rise. This is the fight-or-flight response and it can save your life in a dangerous situation, but it's not helpful if you're just navigating a stressful day. Stress triggers impulsive reactions to everyday conditions, so, in effect, it destroys willpower.

According to Kelly McGonigal, author of *The Willpower Instinct*, when stress is high, you can cultivate more self-control through a pause-and-plan response, noticing your usual reactions and intentionally choosing a more empowered one.[2] To incite willpower, McGonigal says, your brain needs to bring your body on board with your goals and halt your impulses.

One of the most powerful ways to do this is to meditate. Meditation activates and thickens your prefrontal cortex, boosting brain power. Even short bouts of meditation are beneficial. Simply sit quietly with your eyes closed for a few minutes and breathe naturally. If you want the help of a meditation app, a few of my favorites are Headspace, Calm, and Insight Timer.

No time to meditate? Just breathe slowly wherever you are. Consciously slow your breath to four counts in and four counts out. Increase the count to six if you can. Doing so boosts your sense of calm and self-control and allows you to respond more mindfully to difficult situations.

Exercise also boosts self-control, and your brain doesn't really care what type you do as long as you're moving. If you simply begin with a short walk three times per week, you'll reap the benefits. Start small and be consistent.

Shift Your Priorities

You have twenty-four hours in every day—1,440 minutes. If we subtract seven hours for slumber, that leaves us with about one thousand waking minutes to make the most of. Are you using your time wisely?

How we spend our time can be summed up in four categories—obligations, growth, distraction and deception, and waste tasks. The necessity and urgency of each type of task are weighted differently. As you read the descriptions that follow, note which category you spend the bulk of your time in, and pay attention to the specific tasks that get the greatest amount of your attention. Notice your habits around distraction and deception and waste tasks, as we fritter away a lot of time and energy on these. Your goal is to shift your priorities away from those areas so you do more of the things that will bring you success.

Obligations

As a hardworking, contributing member of society you will spend the lion's share of your waking hours tending to obligations: the tasks you have to do every day to live your life with minimal chaos. Obligations include your paid work, along with taking care of your family, your aging parents, and your bills. They also include emergency circumstances and pressing deadlines. If you have an important meeting, it takes precedence over going for a run. If you have a "drop deadline" on a project at work, it comes before dinner out with friends. If the school calls because your child is sick or injured, you stop whatever you're doing and go to them. If you don't take care of these obligations, life will become chaotic, but if obligation rules all your time, you may need to make some changes.

Growth

In an ideal world, when we've met our obligations for the day, we'd all jump into tackling our growth tasks. They include those big, game-changing goals you have for your health, happiness, and career. Everything is this category will help you get ahead personally and professionally. Personal growth tasks include exercise, eating right, getting enough rest, finding better life balance, enjoying leisure time with family and friends, traveling, learning a new hobby, and saving more money. Professional growth tasks include business development, taking a course, returning to school, creative work, organizing your desk or systems, and financial and business planning. If it will help you get ahead personally and professionally, it is a growth task.

Spending time on growth tasks is always a good idea because when you do, not only will you experience personal and professional growth, you'll also lighten the load of obligation. Yet so often tasks in this category remain undone. These tasks bring out your Dreamer. You want to achieve a goal and you believe that you can do the tasks to achieve it, but you can't seem to find the discipline. And then, with the best of intentions, you say, *I'll get to it when...*

Distraction and deception

As you search for more discipline, look closely at the tasks that fall into this category. These are low-priority, ever-present tasks like unimportant emails, phone calls, and "to-dos." You jump to them because you think they'll take only a moment and they're usually easier than the high-priority tasks of growth. They distract you from your goals. These tasks disguise themselves as work, and can fool you into believing you're being productive when you're not. In reality, while these tasks need to get done, there's no hurry. Deception also rears its ugly head when someone's emergency becomes your urgency—for example, when you say yes to requests for your time, even if the tasks are not in your job description, or when your schedule and commitments really need you to say no, but instead you help someone else with a lesser-priority task.

If you spend too much time on distraction and deception tasks, you'll slow your progress. You'll end up using your best energy and time for low-priority tasks, and when it comes to growth tasks, you'll have little left to give.

Waste

Let's face it, we all sometimes need to sit, stare into space, and tune out—but the hours you spend on time wasters, such as excessive television, social media, non-work-related internet, video games, and the like, will impact your efforts to grow. Because of the supercomputer at our fingertips, we waste far more time than ever before. Everything we do in this category feeds 21st-and-a-quarter-century stress. If you tell yourself you don't have time for exercise or other good things, check in with how much time you spend doing waste tasks.

Get to Growth

Your goal is to get to growth. I sometimes call growth tasks the "I'll-get-to-it-when" tasks, since busyness invariably pulls you away from them to tend to the fires lit in obligation and distraction and deception. Those tasks always seem more urgent. Then, once the fires are out, you're likely to drop onto the sofa and do waste tasks because you're too tired to exercise or do any of the other fun and important items in growth. To improve your discipline for the tasks in growth, remember this: you have to act on those tasks; they won't act on you. Where obligation and distraction and deception draw you in by default, you have to consciously plan to get to growth.

Take a few moments to do an inventory of how you spend your time. Which of your growth tasks need more of your attention? Identify them and see if you can move a couple of them to obligation so they become a non-negotiable part of your week. Then, check out some of the following discipline hacks that will help you engage your #SuccessEnergy.

Think big, go small

Dreaming big is good, but if you're overwhelmed by the enormity of the goal in front of you, discipline will tank. You must reframe. Don't overthink whether you can do it or how hard it will be, just break your big goal down into smaller tasks and take the first step. Here are two truths about the tasks we want to accomplish but endlessly procrastinate: (1) it's not the *doing* that's tough, it's getting to it; and (2) *doing* on any level is better than *thinking* about going big.

Go small so you go. Once you start, momentum will carry you forward and you'll keep at it, likely for longer than you planned.

Manage distractions

When you try to do the work, what usually sidetracks your efforts? If you truly hope to accomplish a goal, you have to create an environment that will allow you to do that. If you need to hit a deadline, shut off notifications on your devices so you can have complete focus without interruption. If you're trying to complete a project but the latest game on your phone distracts you too often, remove it from your device. In fact, shut off your device altogether. If you keep getting interrupted when you try to work, put a sign on your door that says: "I am under a tight deadline and will be 100 percent unavailable until 2 p.m. today." Let people know when they can reconnect with you, or whom they can speak to instead. If you're hoping to establish a decent bedtime but Netflix always sucks you in, don't turn it on in the first place. Even better, if that damn television in your bedroom regularly delays your sleep, get it out of there. If you want to eat healthier, don't bring junk foods into your house.

Acknowledge your shortcomings, and don't fool yourself into thinking you can control them *this time*. If they've been a problem before, they'll continue to be a problem until you do something about them.

Control your sensory environment

Our five senses—hearing, touch, sight, smell, and taste—can operate as sneaky distractions if we don't manage them. These senses are naturally triggered all day long, and sometimes they can stop you from doing your best work. Consider how the following affect you:

- **SOUND DISTRACTIONS:** hallway chatter, nearby music or phone conversations, the buzzing light above your desk, or the noisy air conditioner

- **TOUCH DISTRACTIONS:** an uncomfortable chair, an itchy sweater, uncomfortable shoes, or a gritty desktop

- **SIGHT DISTRACTIONS:** anything that comes into your view that draws your focus, like wallpaper or wall hangings, the view from your desk, the quality of your computer screen, or a lack of natural light or windows

- **SMELL DISTRACTIONS:** the aroma of coffee or food, exhaust or paint fumes, bodily odors, perfumes or fragrant products, pets

- **TASTE DISTRACTIONS:** aftertaste, bad breath, whatever you're eating or chewing

Identify which sensory distractions impact your focus, and when you need to do your best work, do it in a place where there will be as few of them as possible.

I find it easy to work in a bustling coffee shop, because the white noise helps me focus, and the smell of coffee (and the cup I'm sipping) keeps me energized. You might find it easier to work in a quiet library or an empty board room, but whatever you do, don't keep working in an area that overloads your senses and undermines your performance.

Change your mind about willpower

Most of us wish we had more willpower. The thing is, your beliefs determine the amount of willpower you possess, and you have more ability to regulate willpower than you think. A Stanford University study showed that participants who believed a person doesn't run out of willpower performed better on tasks than those who viewed willpower as limited.[3] The level of the participants' conviction around either view of willpower coincided with their ability to stick to goals. Participants who believed willpower was finite were more prone to procrastination.

What if you simply decide that you're capable? Square your shoulders, choose to access some of your unlimited willpower, and give yourself an extra hit of motivation for doing the work.

Don't give your power hours to throw-aways

We all have hours in the day when we get our best work done. I call them "power hours" because that's when you will do more work—and better-quality work—than at any other time. For many people, the first couple of hours of the day, when the brain is fresh and the body is re-energized from sleep, are most productive. A night owl's power hours may not begin until after nine in the evening, but when they get going, watch out. And many teenagers do better work in late morning or midday, when their growing, hormone-laden bodies finally wake up.

Identify your power hours, then protect that time for high-priority work, not throw-away tasks like checking email or sorting bills or organizing your desk. If your power hours are at the start of the workday, it can be tempting to ease in by checking email and doing away with quick, low-priority tasks, but why waste your best energy on the minutiae? Instead, take the first few minutes of your day to list the top three high-priority tasks to accomplish that day, and begin on the first one while energy is high, and time is abundant.

Set a timer

If you want to get something done, create a deadline. When you have lots of time to finish a task, you'll invariably waste much of it on distractions and low-priority work, then rush at the last minute to complete the task. When you set a timer, you create a sense of urgency. The length of time you choose will be dependent on the task at hand, but shorter is usually better for focus.

The Pomodoro Technique—a time management method developed by Francesco Cirillo in the 1990s—suggests twenty-five-minute work intervals, followed by five minutes of rest.[4] If you know you have only twenty-five minutes to get the job done, you'll lean in and focus until the timer goes off. If the task isn't done when the timer goes off, take that five-minute break, then set the timer for a second work stint. After four cycles, take a longer break. You can accomplish remarkable results when you introduce a bit of urgency into your work. Seeing how much you can accomplish in short, timed work intervals can also be quite motivating.

Reward yourself

We all like rewards. They make us feel good about what we've accomplished, and they can also motivate us when the work gets tough. Consider these three aspects of worthwhile rewarding:

Timing

How often will you reward your progress? Will you celebrate monthly or based on milestones? Determine frequency ahead of time to work through challenges, and don't simply reward yourself because you feel you need it.

Appropriateness

Your reward needs to be proportionate to the achievement. A two-week vacation after one week of sticking to your plan is an off-balance reward. A day off might be more appropriate. And the reward shouldn't weaken the goal. If your goal is to lose ten pounds and the reward is ice cream, you might want to rethink the reward.

Meaningfulness

Choose rewards that are meaningful to you. If you choose something that feels insignificant, it's not going to have the desired effect. Sometimes the most meaningful reward is the endorphin hit you get when you check that item off your to-do list.

MAKE YOUR rewards fun and creative. Choose rewards that bring you joy without guilt or regret: Treat yourself to a meal at a restaurant you've always wanted to try. Make yourself a fun, personalized certificate, then post it where you can see it every day. Give yourself a longer break—go for a walk or have coffee with a friend. Post your win on social media. Buy yourself some gold stars, create a progress chart, and earn your way to each star. Call a loved one to share about your accomplishment. Take a nap. Take a day off.

Know that it's not meant to be easy

Anything worth having asks you to stretch outside your comfort zone. If the goal feels easy, it probably isn't big enough. The path to success will at times feel very uncomfortable. Get over it. Know that it's not meant to be easy, then do it anyway. Do it because you can, even if you don't feel like it—because you'll rarely feel like it. Do it for no other reason than to prove it to yourself, and because you will step closer to your goal if you take action. Do it to be done with it. Then check that item off your list, celebrate that you no longer need to do it, and get on to the next item.

I'll say it again: if you want success at anything, the effort you put in is worth so much more than any natural gift or talent. To get what you want, you just have to do the freakin' work. And yes, sometimes that road to success will feel like an endless uphill battle. But if you commit to even small amounts of time on the things that matter, you'll make progress, you'll find motivation, and you'll keep going. Strengthen the work ethic and habits that align with your goals and be ready when the momentum of your efforts starts to pull you toward success. It will happen, and I promise you, it will be wonderful.

Engage Your #SuccessEnergy: Discipline Yourself

This chapter has provided a lot of food for thought about discipline, so take a few moments to think about how you hold yourself back from doing your best work. Be honest about the distractions that eat up your time, or the time wasters that use up your energy, and think about small changes you can make, starting today, to work better and with more focus. Consider your personal and professional goals, and answer these questions:

> What do you want that you are not achieving?
> What must you do that you are not yet doing?
> What gets in the way?
> What is your first step toward better?

9

ENERGY AS A MAGIC MULTIPLIER OF SUCCESS

---

66 Energy and persistence
conquer all things. 99

BENJAMIN FRANKLIN

S0 FAR, IN this exploration of The Success-Energy Equation, we've discovered why it's important to set worthwhile goals (G) and write them down. We've explored self-belief (B) and its impact on success, and how both goals and belief feed our discipline (D) to do the work. We've looked at ways to strengthen discipline so we can stay the course longer and reach our goals sooner. And we've discussed how 21st-and-a-quarter-century stress, if left unchecked, can hinder progress with G, B, and D. Now we're going to talk about how energy (E) improves not only our health and longevity, but also so many other determinants of success.

I've spent most of my life in the realm of human performance —as a competitive kayaker, avid outdoor enthusiast, mountain biker, rock climber, and snowboarder. I am a psychology major turned kinesiology master. I've worked as a college instructor, health educator, and personal trainer, always interested in what makes people tick, inside and out. As a coach, consultant, and professional speaker, I travel all over North America to educate busy, driven professionals about purpose, productivity, and the pursuit of better. I've spent most of my career talking about health and energy management, and the power it gives us to do everything better. The information I share isn't earth-shattering or mind-blowing; it's everyday, unsexy, I-don't-have-time-for-it health and energy management. I present it in a fun and enlightening way that hopefully helps people learn *why* care of body and mind should remain a priority, especially when 21st-and-a-quarter-century stress is bearing down on you.

In chapter 2, I began the conversation about health as a driver for success and listed three reasons why, on the path to success, energy and health management is so important: increased quality of life, increased quality of success, and increased probability of success. These are worthwhile reasons for having health and energy management as part of your success plan, but I'm going to remind you of a fourth: that ever-invasive, distracting, pervasive 21st-and-a-quarter-century stress that overloads our bandwidth and hinders progress with goals, belief, and discipline can best be managed with remarkably simple health and energy strategies.

When you think about improving your energy, my guess is that you look at how much exercise you're getting, the quality and length of your sleep, and the foods you eat. Attention to physical health is essential for sustained, productive energy, but there are two other ways to boost energy that are less obvious and equally critical: mental/cognitive recovery and emotional connection.

These key energy management strategies—recovery, connection, and health—will not only reduce the impact that 21st-and-a-quarter-century stress has on your G, B, and D, they'll also increase the physical, mental, emotional, and cognitive capacity within you to drive your success to new heights. I've said it before: the key is in E, and it's how your body works to help you work better.

Get Energized by Recovery

"Hard work pays off." "The early bird gets the worm." "Winners never quit." Most of us have heard statements like these throughout our lives. We've been raised to believe that if we want success the only way to achieve it is to put our head down, work long hours, and be available 24/7. Hard work will be rewarded, right?

Although success requires that you work hard, these days, with life coming at us from every direction and with digital noise filling all available downtime, if you want success it may be just as important to *recover* hard. High-performance athletes understand this better than most. To succeed at a high level in sport, they must work hard at training, and then allow their bodies to adequately recover so the effects of training can take hold. Without proper recovery, athletes struggle with injuries, excessive fatigue, and loss of enthusiasm for their sport because of over-training. That won't bring results.

In 2001, in a pivotal *Harvard Business Review* article, Jim Loehr and Tony Schwartz introduced the concept of the corporate athlete and the idea that if individuals want to enjoy a long career while driving toward high levels of excellence, they need to train with the precision, focus, and adaptability of a professional athlete.[1] Through decades of research with elite athletes, Loehr and Schwartz noted that successful professional athletes spend 90 percent of their time training so that they can perform at a high level 10 percent of the time. They embrace optimal nutrition, sleep, psychological support, and rest. Depending on the sport, their off-season—a time used for mental, physical, and emotional recovery—may span anywhere from two to five months per year.

By comparison, average corporate professionals might spend 90 percent of their time performing, and 10 percent training. They'll work long hours under high stress, they'll eat poorly, skip breaks, and forgo sleep. Their "off-season" might include a couple of weeks of holidays and a handful of long weekends, during which they'll check emails and connect with the office. And they will likely work forty or fifty years with no significant breaks.

Looked at this way, it seems absurd that common professional culture is so accepting of skipped breaks and working lunches, not to mention after-hours emails. In truth, many successful organizations bank on the hard work of their employees, so much so that they'll create an inviting, fun office environment that might include game rooms, nap pods, comfortable modern work spaces, chef-run kitchens where food is free, and access to massage therapists and fitness facilities. You might be thinking, "I'd like to work in a place like that!" but unless the organization values rest and recovery for its employees, these perks simply make it convenient to work long hours. With all these amenities, why would you need to leave?

Stewart Butterfield, the co-founder and CEO of online team workspace Slack, has a different take on productivity. The company motto is "work hard and go home." Having lived and preached the sixty-hour work week culture in his early career, Butterfield now understands that people have lives outside work, and when his employees have freedom to design their own work-life balance, they are a motivated and happy workforce. Employees at Slack have a flexible work schedule and are encouraged to take time off to enjoy exciting adventures. New parents get ample parental leave. Additionally, their offices are beautiful, welcoming spaces that bring the outdoors in. They're also designed for productivity, not play, so employees can work hard and go home. Since it launched in 2009, Slack has grown to be worth more than $20 billion, so it appears they are onto something.

Work Hard and Recover

If you want to do your best work and sustain it over time, if you want to embrace the discipline of a corporate athlete along with all the hard work, allow your body and mind adequate short- and long-term recovery so your efforts can be sustained at a high level. Our tech-fed, digitally distracted, 21st-and-a-quarter-century-stress-filled existence demands it.

Amazingly, implementing recovery into your success plan is relatively simple, as long as you listen to your body. It knows what it needs, and when you provide what it asks for, body *and* mind will answer in kind. If you've been working so hard that you're burned out and uninspired, recovery might mean several weeks off or a change or reduction in workload. That can be difficult to do, but the good news is, you can gain significant energy and bandwidth by simply tuning in to the signs your body sends you.

General, ever-present fatigue is a sign that should not be ignored. Amp up your sleep routine and try some of the physical-health energizers that follow. During your workday, note when any of these signs start to affect your productivity: loss of focus, wandering mind, distraction, fidgetiness, absent-mindedness, sleepiness, or yawning. You may also feel hungry or need the restroom. These are all messages from your body telling you it needs a break. You'll often experience one or more of them after ninety minutes of focused work. Stop what you're doing and then try a couple of these renewal strategies:

- Stand up and stretch. Walk around your office. Do jumping jacks.

- Take a longer break. In fact, take regular breaks, especially if you're working on tasks that require mental focus. When you do, go tech-free, and get outside for a bit of movement and fresh air.

- Eat lunch away from your desk as much as possible. Instead of depending on your smartphone for company, ask a friend to join you, read a good book, or listen to music.

- Fuel your body and mind with regular snacks and hydrating H_2O.

- When stress mounts, stop and breathe deeply and slowly for a couple of minutes.

- Incorporate movement into your work. Stand up for phone calls. Walk while you're processing ideas. Try walking meetings.

- Nap if you need to, or seek out a quiet room to just sit and rest your brain.

After a particularly intense work session or meeting, take a longer mental break, like going for a walk or a workout. Or implement one or more of the ideas I just listed. If you habitually weave recovery strategies into your daily routine, your energy will sustain you through the workday.

Every day, as you leave work and before you go home, determine a decompression strategy that will allow you to shift from work mode to relax mode, to shut off work for even a short period of time. Go to the gym on your way home, listen to music you love on your commute, sit and breathe silently in your vehicle, go for a walk at a park nearby. Do something that frees you from technology and helps you get present to your non-work surroundings and the people in it. Then, when you get home, put your phone away, smile, and be fully present to your family, your pets, or simply to yourself. After a stressful, busy day it may be tempting to hit the sofa and binge-watch your favorite shows until bedtime, but that may not be the best use of your downtime. Recovery strategies outside work are almost as important as those you implement during your work-day, perhaps as a reminder that life is not meant to be all about work. In chapter 4, I shared twelve ways to move from autopilot to awareness. In the fight against 21st-and-a-quarter-century stress and burnout, every one of those ideas can double as recovery strategies. Flip to page 70 for a quick reminder, then add a few to your daily plan.

The ongoing relaxation and recovery you need to be at your best will also be influenced by the other two energizers: connection and health.

Get Energized by Connection

When energy is low, you're more likely to caffeinate than converse, but science suggests that the latter—human connection—is a worthwhile physical, mental, and emotional energizer. So, if you need a boost of energy, spend some time with people you like.

Your brain is an inherently social organ, designed to help you interact with others and form strong relationships. For our ancestors, those bonds contributed to their survival and well-being as they worked together to build shelter, hunt and gather, and keep predators at bay. Today the same is true, although the stressors have changed. People who feel more connected to others experience lower levels of anxiety and depression.[2] Strong social connection helps you strengthen your immune system and recover from disease faster, and you may even live longer.[3] Studies also show that when you feel connected to others, you have higher self-esteem, greater empathy for others, and are more trusting and cooperative, which leads others to be more trusting and cooperative toward you.[4] When you spend time with people you like, your body releases the hormone oxytocin, which contributes to relaxation, trust, and psychological stability.[5]

Scientists have long held that, as humans, we have an innate need for belonging, which if not met can in extreme cases impact people's ability to follow rules, regulate behavior, and contribute positively to society.[6] And our need for interaction won't be met by connecting with our online "friends." Indeed, it could be argued that our device addiction has served only to heighten our social isolation and feelings of loneliness. In chapter 4, I shared that British prime minister Theresa May once appointed a minister for loneliness. She did that because she recognized that lonely people—the elderly, their caregivers, people who have lost loved ones, and marginalized groups— often have no one to talk to, and without help can overwhelm the health system.

So, what can you do to strengthen connections and, by association, boost your personal energy? These reminders might help:

- Carve out time with friends and family who fill you up. Reconnect with old friends you value.

- Focus on quality interactions rather than quantity of friends. You will gain more by having one or two close friends to confide in than by maintaining dozens of superficial connections.

- Cultivate connections and social activities that you enjoy best. Intertwining hobbies with social time is a double-win.

- Use social media as a way to make plans offline. If you use social media itself as a destination for connecting—with the exception of pandemic-era necessity, of course—it will only add to social isolation.

- Make regular plans to meet friends for activities like game night, a hike in the mountains, or dinner club. There's nothing better than getting active and social at the same time.

- Stay connected with long-distance loved ones in person or by phone. Even email, social media, or video chat is better than not connecting at all.

- At work, invite colleagues to join you for coffee or lunch. Better yet, exercise together for added energy and accountability.

- Look for opportunities to collaborate on projects that will benefit from ideation. Even a short meet-up to brainstorm can energize social connections *and* the work you are doing.

- As you navigate through your day, do so with head up and eyes open. Greet people, engage in conversation, ask questions, and even ask for help. A smile can go a long way to initiating those connections and brightening everyone's day.

Get Energized by Health

People are often motivated to embark on a health program simply to improve their physical health and appearance. It's not a bad reason, because the benefits are impressive. Regular exercise and healthy eating help control weight, which can prevent obesity and the risk factors associated with it. Plus, we typically feel better about ourselves when we carry less weight. With regular exercise and a healthy diet, we also improve overall health and reduce disease risk with some cancers, diabetes, heart disease, and stroke. Plus, bone density and muscle strength increase, and blood pressure, cholesterol levels, and triglycerides improve.

When you prioritize health, you live longer. Studies show that physical activity can reduce your risk of dying early from many leading causes of death, like heart disease and certain cancers.[7] Good sleep is a part of this, and regular exercise helps us fall asleep faster and stay asleep longer. Overall energy is improved, and stress is reduced. And these two factors combined provide us with a greater capacity to cope.

So many amazing body and mind benefits are packed into every healthful decision. Here are some of the highlights:

Physical health benefits

Better health, lower risk of disease
Longevity
Improved sleep
Improved energy
Weight management

Mental and emotional health benefits

Reduced feelings of anxiety and depression
Lower stress, better capacity to cope with stress
Improved self-confidence, self-esteem, self-efficacy
Improved social interaction
Improved mood

Cognitive health benefits

Improved attention span and focus
Enhanced creativity
Better critical thinking
Better problem solving
Improved memory and learning

THE PURSUIT of health has become a puzzling, irritating, sometimes dangerous obsession for some, which in many ways has the opposite of its intended effect. We're looking for an easy way out of health shortfalls that likely took years to manifest, and there's no quick fix for poor health habits. All the shiny, big-energy, fatigue-busting, digestion-aiding, fat-burning fads have distracted us from what really matters: a clear understanding of the basics of health. You need that, and you need to establish a foundation of sound habits—health trends be damned.

In our busy lives, fitting in even the basics is challenging, so let's keep it simple with four non-negotiables for better health and energy: move more, eat better, prioritize sleep, and stay hydrated—MESH for health. Let's take a deeper look at each of these must-dos to boost your success energy.

Move your body, strengthen your brain

When you move more, not only do you feel better physically, you also improve your *emotional health* in considerable ways. During exercise, your body releases endorphins that can improve your mood and help you feel more relaxed. The positive feelings that arise from even a single session of exercise are known to boost self-esteem, and in the long term, exercise makes you feel better about your physical capabilities and how you look. It also provides you with a sense of accomplishment and boosts confidence and self-efficacy that you can carry into everything you do. When you feel better about yourself you also interact better with others, so social health improves when you move more.

Movement also improves *mental health* in remarkable ways. Regular exercise can reduce anxiety by lessening the reactivity of your brain's fight-or-flight response. Through regular exercise that increases heart rate, anxious people who typically associate rapid heartbeat with an anxiety attack can develop tolerance for those symptoms and mitigate associated stress. Regular exercise can reduce depressive symptoms, and studies have even shown that exercise can be as effective as medication for some, though proper medical care and diagnosis of depression is always recommended.[8] Many studies support that regular exercise can also have a positive influence on anxiety, ADHD, and more. It also reduces stress, helps you sleep better, and boosts your overall mood. Even modest amounts of exercise can make a difference.[9]

Our brains evolved while we were moving, not while sedentary, so it makes sense that exercise would have a profound effect on our cognition. There are so many ways that exercise improves *cognitive health*. Aerobic exercise such as walking, running, or biking raises your heart rate and increases blood flow to your brain. As breathing increases, more oxygen is pumped into your bloodstream and up to your brain. This leads to the production of new neurons in certain parts of your brain that control memory and thinking. This neurogenesis increases brain volume, which is believed to improve cognition and help protect against the effects of dementia.[10]

Exercise also stimulates the production of neurotrophins, proteins that promote the survival and function of neurons.[11] This leads to greater brain plasticity, which enhances memory and learning.[12] If that isn't enough, exercise also increases neurotransmitters in the brain, specifically serotonin and norepinephrine, both of which regulate mood, boost memory, and improve information processing. Your brain remembers more when your body is active.

Research also shows that regular exercisers do better on tests of creativity than their sedentary counterparts. This boost in creativity seems to be linked to improved divergent and convergent thinking, which helps you come up with more ideas and zero in on worthwhile options. Not only does this feed creativity, it also enhances problem solving. And, finally, the endorphins that are released during exercise help you work better once you stop moving. After exercise, your ability to prioritize improves, allowing you to block out distractions and better concentrate on the task at hand. That focus even improves for two to three hours after you've exercised.[13]

I often say that I exercise for my mind and my body reaps the benefits. The mind and body are deeply connected. And while your brain is the command center for your body's movement, the way you move can also affect how you think and feel.

How much is enough?

What type of exercise is the best, and how much is enough? There is no simple answer to this two-part question. The verdict is still out on the ideal exercise dose for boosting cognitive health. Many studies have linked the cognitive improvements following exercise to the increased capacity of the heart, lungs, and blood to transport oxygen. These physiological changes come about largely through aerobic exercises, and experts agree that regular cardiovascular conditioning can improve brain health.[14] Cognitive improvements have also been observed with low-intensity mind-body exercises like tai chi or qigong, both of which focus on breathing and mindful movement, which have been linked to improved brain health.[15]

I believe the most important decision around exercise is not so much *what* you do, but *that* you do. Choose activities you enjoy. Variety is best. At least three days each week, move in ways that increase your heart rate and breathing. You should be breathless but still able to converse. A little sweat is a good thing. Strength train at least once per week too, with weights, yoga, or the like. And any time you have the choice to move more, do it:

- Walk ten minutes to a meeting instead of driving.
- Take the stairs instead of the elevator.
- Get off transit a few stops earlier and walk.
- Park your car a few blocks from your office.
- Drive partway to work, then cycle from there.
- Do crunches during all the commercial breaks while you watch your favorite show.
- Go for a walk after dinner. Take your kids, your spouse, your neighbor, your dog.
- Give your dog an extra walk each day and add hills to the route.
- Do jumping jacks until the kettle boils.
- Do walking lunges down the hallway.
- Run up the stairs. Chasing kids counts.

It doesn't matter if you're a couch potato, a now-and-then exerciser, or an all-out fitness buff. Your goal for movement should be to consistently do more than what is normal for you. Start small if you have to, but start. Remember, our brains evolved during movement, so move more, do it regularly, and feel the positive effects of exercise for brain health.

Exercise for a Business Edge

The next time you try to talk yourself out of exercise because you have too much work to do, think instead of exercise as part of your business strategy. Schedule your exercise for first thing in the morning or during your lunch break, for two reasons:

1   If you schedule exercise before or during your work-day, you are more likely to stick to it because you are

> less likely to be waylaid by late-day emergencies or
> fatigue.
>
> 2 The earlier you get moving, the sooner you can reap the
>   full benefits of the brain boost exercise will give you.
>
> On days where you have an important meeting or pre-
> sentation, plan for a morning walk or run so you're firing
> on all cylinders—mentally, physically, emotionally, *and*
> cognitively—during the meeting.

Eat to Fuel Success

Your brain works hard 24/7 to monitor your thoughts and
movements, regulate your breathing and heartbeat, and fire
up your senses. Because it's always on, your brain is a massively
energy-hungry organ that requires a constant supply of fuel,
which comes from the foods you eat.

You've likely heard the phrase "garbage in, garbage out."
Well, it could not be a truer way to underline the importance
of healthy eating, for body and mind. What you eat directly
affects the structure and function of your brain and, ultimately,
your mood and thought processes. Like an expensive car, your
brain functions best on premium fuel. Fresh, healthy foods that
contain vitamins, minerals, and antioxidants will nourish the
brain and protect it from oxidative stress. Also just like with an
expensive car, your brain health can be compromised if you eat
too much low-grade fuel like processed or refined foods. Many
studies have linked high-sugar diets to impaired brain function and have noted worsening symptoms of mood disorders.[16]
Beyond impairing your body's regulation of insulin, high-sugar

foods also promote inflammation and oxidative stress, which is an imbalance between free radicals and antioxidants that causes tissue damage.[17]

Here's an interesting fact about food that suggests that what you eat may directly influence your mood: the neurotransmitter serotonin helps regulate sleep and appetite, mediate mood, and inhibit pain. About 95 percent of serotonin is produced in your gastrointestinal tract, which is lined with a hundred million nerve cells. It stands to reason then that the inner workings of your digestive system don't just help you digest food, they also guide your emotions. Studies have shown that those who take probiotics that introduce "good" bacteria into the system have reduced anxiety levels, lower perception of stress, and improved mental outlook compared with those who do not.[18] Fermented foods like kimchi, miso, sauerkraut, pickles, or kombucha act as natural probiotics and can be good for your gut health as well.

To fuel a healthy brain, follow a healthy dietary plan that includes lots of fruits, vegetables, legumes, and whole grains. Try to get most protein from plant sources and fish and choose healthy fats, such as olive oil or canola, rather than saturated fats. Although there is no single superfood for your brain, certain foods are particularly rich in healthful components like omega-3 fatty acids, B vitamins, and antioxidants, which are known to support brain health: green leafy vegetables like kale, spinach, or broccoli; fatty fish like salmon, cod, or canned light tuna; berries; and walnuts. If you incorporate these foods into a healthy diet on a regular basis, you can improve your brain health. You can also get a short-term concentration boost from your morning cup of coffee or tea.

Pay attention to how different foods make you feel, not just in the moment, but the next day as well. Try eating a clean diet for a week or two—that means cutting out all processed foods and sugar. Some clean diets also encourage the elimination of flour and dairy for periods of time. It might sound extreme, but how well you can eat without flour, sugar, or dairy may surprise you. Your meals will be high in fruits and vegetables, lean meats, and other proteins, legumes, nuts, and seeds. Admittedly the first day or two can feel like a bit of a detox, but you'll start to feel remarkably good after a few days of sugar- and flour-free eating.

After a couple of weeks, introduce foods back into your diet, one by one, and see how you feel. You may discover that you prefer to minimize certain foods because you feel more energetic and focused without them. When you listen to your body and choose healthy food options to fuel you, you will have more energy to give to your goals, which will amplify your success. Just remember that every one of us has a different nutritional profile, and it's always a great idea to consult with a registered dietician for guidance and sound information.

Sleep to Reset Your System

Sleep has many benefits, including providing energy and helping you feel better, but there's a lot more to it than that. The Division of Sleep Medicine at Harvard Medical School has done a great deal of research on the effects of sleep. Not surprisingly, these studies have shown time and again that sleep plays a key role in promoting physical health, longevity, and emotional well-being.[19] While you sleep, your body uses most of the night to heal damage done to your cells and tissues. It pumps out proteins to repair cells, and growth hormones to promote muscle development. The glymphatic system flushes the toxins from your brain to help clarify your thoughts and consolidate your memories.

Make no mistake, sleep deprivation eventually affects every aspect of your daily life. Inadequate rest impairs your ability to think, handle stress, maintain a healthy immune system, and moderate your emotions. Research has shown that, in general, people would be happier, healthier, and safer if they were to sleep an extra sixty to ninety minutes per night.[20] While a tiny percentage of the population does fine on little sleep, those people are incredibly rare. Most of us need seven to nine hours. And 40 percent of us aren't getting it.

If you regularly get jolted out of sleep by your alarm and then zombie through your day, you'd do well to focus on improving the quality and quantity of your sleep. Chronic sleep deprivation can lead to anxiety, irritability, depression, hypertension, obesity, type 2 diabetes, and deficiencies in reaction time, creativity, critical thinking, and problem solving.

Although many benefits of sleep are obvious, there are also many lesser-known advantages of quality slumber. Here are just a few of them.

Perk up your mood

Inadequate sleep affects your judgment, increases agitation, and muddies your mood. Most of us can navigate the occasional sleeplessness-induced grumpy spell, but chronic sleep deficiency can lead to serious mood disorders like anxiety or depression.

Improve your memory

Fatigue negatively impacts concentration and memory. The more tired you become, the more difficulty you will have recalling incidents, lessons, faces, and facts. The good news is that while you sleep, the filing cabinets in your brain have time to organize, imprint the day's new knowledge, and improve your memory. If you often forget the details, *sleeping on it* may help.

Boost your energy

Who doesn't feel more energized and alert after a good night's sleep? You can use that short-term energy to boost your long-term energy. Take your invigorated body outdoors. Engage with your surroundings and be active. You'll sleep better again that night and gain even more energy.

Reduce your stress

Sleep is a necessary function to help manage the physical effects of stress. And since 21st-and-a-quarter-century stress is pervasive, we need to prioritize sleep more than ever. The relationship between stress and sleep can be a self-propelling cycle, because stress often gets in the way of quality sleep, and sleep is one of the main ways to effectively minimize stress.

FOR QUALITY sleep, part of the answer lies in your pre-sleep routine. You won't fall into blissful sleep if you race through a hectic day and then overstimulate your mind with high-intensity television, blast your brain cells with internet information overload, or keep working until lights out. And your body also won't wind down well if you feed it unhealthy snacks or too much food or alcohol right before bed. Improve the quality and quantity of your sleep by developing a pre-sleep routine that will help you doze off more quickly. Here are a few tips:

- Start winding down at least thirty minutes before you want to sleep.

- Avoid fatty or high-protein foods before bed. Your body has to work harder to digest them, so they may keep you awake.

- Cut out TV, internet, and computer time before bed to avoid an overstimulated bed-brain.

- Read or take a bath.

- Stretch or meditate.

- Sip a cup of non-caffeinated tea.

- Keep your room cool (about 18°C or 64°F), dark, and clean.

- Use a comfy pillow that suits your sleep style, plus cozy sheets and pajamas.

- If possible, make sure your bed provides you the right type of support.

Hydrate for Energy and Clarity

Simply put, hydration boosts brain power. Over 60 percent of an adult human body is water, and every system in the body depends on proper hydration, including the brain and nervous system. Water is the second most important nutrient for the human body, following oxygen, and although you can go without food for a few weeks, you won't last more than three or four days without water.

Your brain is 75 percent water, so water is an essential element in neurological transmissions. According to University of Texas neuroscientist Joshua Gowin, brain cells require a delicate balance between water and other elements to operate.[21] All of your thinking is helped along by little zaps in your brain, but when you're dehydrated, that balance is disrupted and your brain loses efficiency. Mild dehydration may be present with just a 1 to 2 percent drop in body water, and research has shown that lack of water to the brain can impair short-term memory function and the recall of long-term memory.[22] It can also cause headaches, brain fog, exhaustion, sleep issues, stress, anger, depression, and other symptoms.

Lack of water is the number one trigger of daytime fatigue. Dehydration can very quickly sap your energy. Even mild dehydration can lead to fatigue, muscle weakness, dizziness, and other symptoms that will affect your productivity and enthusiasm for your work.

Believe it or not, no single water intake recommendation fits everyone. Common wisdom is to drink eight eight-ounce glasses of water every day (two liters). Sip early and sip often. Your body will tell you when it's better hydrated—if only by the number of trips you need to take to the restroom!

Here are three questions to ask yourself to support hydration every day:

Am I thirsty?

This may seem obvious, but if you're thirsty I don't want you to ignore it. If you're already thirsty, it's too late. You're heading toward dehydration, so it's situation critical to top up on those hydrating fluids.

What color is my pee?

Yeah, you read correctly. To stay hydrated, you need to become a bowl watcher. Once you're done with number one, look at the color of your pee. If it's dark yellow and has a strong odor, you haven't been drinking enough water. If you have been drinking enough water, your urine will be light yellow or clear in color. Nice work! Pay attention to volume as well. If you don't produce much urine throughout the day and it's dark in color, you likely need more fluids. Note, however, that if you take B vitamins, your pee will be bright yellow.

How am I feeling?

If you feel light-headed and tired, unable to concentrate, or are experiencing frequent headaches, pay attention! These could be signs that you're dehydrated.

WE'VE COME full-circle on my Success-Energy Equation—
$S = G \times f(B,D)^E$—where success (S) equals setting clear, exciting
goals (G), having belief (B) in yourself regarding those goals,
and the discipline (D) to do the work. And now you can see more
clearly how all these variables are influenced by the energy
(E) within. And not just through exercise and eating right.

As you think about health and energy management in your
own life, pay attention to how you move, eat, sleep, and hydrate,
for sure, but don't forget about vital recovery tactics and how
important it is to connect with others. Health, recovery, and
connection: they all drive your #SuccessEnergy in powerful
ways, and through the ideas I've shared in this chapter I hope
you better understand why each should be a non-negotiable
part of your own success formula.

Engage Your #SuccessEnergy:
Small Steps to an Energetic Life

We have covered a lot of ground for prioritizing personal energy
that will drive success. Now it's time to establish your new-and-
improved health and energy management plan. Remember
that small steps are worthwhile, especially when taken daily.

First, what are you already doing well? What health and energy practices are you proud of and do you plan to continue?

Which energy-draining habits would you like to reduce or
eliminate?

Finally, what new ideas will you incorporate into a re-
energized energy management strategy? Don't forget to
consider recovery tactics and social connection along with
health strategies.

10

THE SUCCESS-ENERGY CONNECTION

---

66 Slowing down is a power move. 99

AMY CUDDY

I**N THE MONTHS** leading up to the completion of the first draft of this book, my life was over-the-top busy. Not only was I trying to write in my spare time, but between April and December I also flew somewhere to present every single week. Because I was traveling so much, I taught very few of the cycle classes that normally keep me fit and energized. Sure, I'd hit the hotel gyms when I could, but my exercise sessions on the road were invariably shorter and less intense than my classes at my gym, and I wasn't doing any weight training. I attempted to eat healthfully during my travels, but that didn't always go well either. The weight was inching on and my energy was decreasing.

Between trips I would unpack, do laundry, and repack for the next week's travel. Then I would be chained to my desk, trying to catch up on any paperwork and preparation that wasn't possible on the road. I also had housework to do, coaching clients and cycle classes to fit in, and social visits to catch up on, not to mention finding quality time with my also-busy hubby. I was grumpy, always tired, and definitely on autopilot a lot during that busy stretch.

While I was on one of my business trips, our beloved eleven-year-old dog, Lilly, took a sudden turn with her health, and my husband and I made the very difficult decision to have her euthanized before I returned home. That was one of the most heartbreaking decisions I've ever had to be a part of, and I felt the emotional strain of it for months. Her loss filled me with such sadness, and only added to the emotional and physical energy drain I already felt.

Right after I delivered my last presentation of the year, I rushed to send the first draft of this book to my editor, then I hopped on another plane and headed to a professional speakers association convention that was being held across the country. I normally look forward to this annual event because I get to connect with dear colleagues, talk about the business of speaking, and learn ways to grow my business, and we always have a lot of fun.

This year, though, given the schedule I had been keeping and the fatigue I was feeling, this convention was the last place I wanted to be. Besides, a day and a half after I got back from the convention, my husband and I were leaving for a monthlong trip to New Zealand. I should have been looking forward to that adventure, but because there was still so much left to prepare for the trip, I wasn't. Suffice it to say I was feeling burned out and overwhelmed.

It's ironic, because I was writing a book about how your body works to help you work better and how health and energy are key to overall success, yet despite knowing better, I had let my own health and energy take a back seat to my schedule and circumstances. As I flew to the convention it dawned on me that I had inadvertently become a subject in my own case study. "Interesting," I said to myself. "Now what?"

Although I didn't catch up on sleep while at the convention, I spent those four days largely disconnected from email, social media, and the internet, and instead connected with my colleagues. My schedule was no longer insane, and I didn't think about work or the manuscript. I just enjoyed a lot of chats (and a lot of hugs) with great people, attended some fantastic sessions, laughed endlessly with my Mastermind gals, fit a couple of exercise sessions in, and spent a night dancing at our gala event. I left the conference feeling tired but refreshed, because I'd shifted gears in a way that would allow my brain to slow down and process everything that had happened in the last eight months.

Before I left for the convention, I had rushed to complete the book manuscript to meet a self-imposed deadline. I wanted to leave for New Zealand and not have to worry about writing. On the flight home, however, I started thinking about that damn manuscript because now, with a few days away from it and a clear head to process it, I knew I needed to make some changes to the sections of the book I'd rushed to finish. In the months I was writing in earnest, I had been so close to the content that I had grown sick and tired of looking at it. It was as if all the words were tangled together in my head. And I'd been so busy in the rest of my life, neglecting my health and forgoing fun, that I was too frazzled to realize that my foggy brain wasn't doing its best work.

Isn't it interesting that a little downtime and connection with others—a small shift away from the 21st-and-a-quarter-century stress that was bearing down on me—gave my brain just enough of an energy boost to help me see clearly again? When I got home, I emailed my editor and my project manager, shared my epiphany with them, and said I needed more time. I told them I would try to do the rewrites during our holiday, but even as I typed those words I felt my stress levels rise and realized that probably wouldn't happen.

I was still tired and burned out from the chaos of the last several months. I needed this time away to restore my energy. I needed time with my husband to reconnect. We deserved unencumbered time together to explore New Zealand, to mountain bike, golf, drink wine, and spend time with friends. We'd been planning and saving for this trip for almost two years, so I *really* didn't want to work while we were away. So, I didn't. I allowed common sense to prevail. I listened to what my mind and body were telling me they needed.

Instead, on the fourteen-hour flight from Vancouver to Auckland, I talked with my husband about the ideas I had for the book rewrites, and as he shared insights and we discussed concepts and changes, I took copious notes... while sipping gin and tonic. In New Zealand we caught up on sleep and napped when we wanted to; we ate good food and drank good wine; we explored new places, had many adventures, and had fun with good friends. We walked every day and mountain biked *a lot*, sometimes riding for three hours or more, and during these active times I often found my mind wandering to the book. I made notes many evenings, but I didn't pull out my laptop. We enjoyed the holiday completely work-free and loved every minute of it.

I returned home energized, refreshed, and truly excited to get back to work. The stressful months that led up to our holiday were a good reminder for me that no matter how crazy life gets, no matter how seemingly important the deadline or how busy the schedule, if you want to be at your productive best, it's vital to prioritize physical, mental, and emotional health, no matter what. It's how we work. Science says so, and yet I so flagrantly ignored the studies *and* my own good advice. Yup, even when we know better, common sense sometimes needs a kick in the ass.

With a clear head and a renewed enthusiasm for my book, I completed the rewrites in ten days and then recommitted to my self-care. I wanted to maintain the health and vitality that followed me home from our trip, so I relaunched my cycle classes and added a strength class to my teaching schedule. I reminded myself that exercise should not be up for negotiation, because when I do it regularly, I work better. The same is true of sleep, so I committed to an earlier bedtime and better sleep hygiene, especially during the week. That regimen includes less alcohol, a cool bedroom, a weighted comforter on our bed, and pink noise before bed to calm my mind and induce deeper sleep. My husband and I are also trying to eat cleaner meals, which for us means leaner meats, less pasta and bread, and more veggies, fruits, and salads. It feels good to make these small changes and we definitely feel better.

Through my accidental personal case study, I regained focus and recharged my life, and it really helped me get shit done. I reconnected with not only *how* I work but also *why* it matters. I'm simply happier, healthier, and more productive when I give my mind and body what they need.

So, how about you? What are your mind and body asking for, and are you listening?

At the very start of this book, I suggested that the world we live in is demanding more from us than ever before—because of technology, crazy traffic, busy schedules, 24/7 connectedness, non-stop in-your-face news and world events, and the stress of it all—and that perhaps we need a different way to deal with it: a move toward simplicity, and a prioritization of health and energy management to rise above the noise and help drive success. I hope you're encouraged by the simplicity of some of my ideas.

You'll also recall that I said you can get by without energy. You can get by without taking care of your health, managing your stress, or tending to your relaxation needs. You can find success even if you eat poorly, smoke, drink too much, sleep poorly, don't exercise, have no life balance, and maintain high stress. I hope this book has provided a worthwhile argument for why you shouldn't. If you truly want to live a happy, healthy, successful life, inattention to health and energy management simply doesn't make sense.

As you've read through each chapter, you've gained ideas and information not only to address 21st-and-a-quarter-century stress, but also to strengthen your physical, emotional, mental, and cognitive capacities in simple but effective ways. Implement those ideas and keep at them, because the more you do, the more equipped you will be to knock down those internal and external barriers that block your way to success.

$$S = G \times f(B,D)^E$$

Work the equation. As the energy within you increases, you'll feel great about yourself and set bigger, more focused goals that you'll be more excited to chase. Belief in yourself will run through everything that you do. Self-doubt will lessen, and personal resolve will increase. You'll begin to look at your goals not only as tasks you can conquer but also as outcomes that you deserve. Why not you? Why not more? Why not now?

That's The Success-Energy Equation, and it's a formula worth calculating!

Engage Your #SuccessEnergy: Seize the Freakin' Day

You've just finished reading a book about how to find success at higher levels, and hopefully you're excited by the ideas I've shared. To help you make the most of what you've learned, I want to leave you with one final tactic that is so anchored in common sense, I don't know why we don't do it more often.

Begin.

Take action in one significant way today on something that will drive your dreams forward. It doesn't even matter if the step is small, because movement creates momentum, and momentum feeds motivation. Begin, and then do it again tomorrow, and the next day, and the one after that, until the results get you excited to keep going.

I've said it before: it's not *doing* it that's tough, it's *getting to it,* and small efforts at action are better than big thoughts never realized. So, before you go, jot down your answers to these "take action" questions, then get out there and engage your newfound #SuccessEnergy!

What's the first thing you will do to get the ball rolling on your plans?

How might you carve out a bit of time every day to take the next step?

How will you track your progress and celebrate accomplishments?

Carpe Freakin' Diem!

ACKNOWLEDGMENTS

MOST AUTHORS WILL agree that by the time a book gets to the completion phase, months—more like years— have passed, and it becomes a nerve-wracking task to think back to *all* the people who influenced, guided, supported, or helped in some small or significant way to bring a book to life. I'm blessed to have a lot of difference-makers in my life.

I'll start with my coaching clients and audiences, who shine a light on the challenges we all face and guide me toward the problems I can help them solve. I'm inspired to do the work I do because of you, and I love my job.

There are two people who unknowingly provided me with inspiration for this book. My speaker buddy Gair Maxwell, while reviewing one of my presentations, gave me the idea for the title of this book. At first, I developed a keynote with the same name, and soon realized there was a book in there. My friend, mentor, and speaker coach, Toni Newman, encouraged me to develop my own proprietary programs and has always inspired me to think bigger and do better. Some of the ideas we worked on together many years ago provide the framework for my Success-Energy Equation today, and often as I wrote, her voice was in my head pushing me to work at an idea until, "Oooo, I just got goosebumps!" I love you, Toni!

My friend Nancy Loraas and I meet almost weekly to talk about writing, coaching, business, and life in general. Her enthusiastic encouragement and support of this book fueled me on the days when I didn't feel like writing, or if I was beating myself up for taking so long to finish the damn book. She has been a great sounding board for my ideas and championed many aspects of the book before I saw the true worth of my words. Thank you, Nancy.

My assistant Tanya Koob painstakingly formatted every citation at the end of this book, freeing up my time to work on edits and other tasks. She also kept asking me, "How's the book coming?" because she's been patiently waiting to be able to share it with my clients. Share away, Tanya!

To my gals Tina Varughese, Lisa Vlooswyk, and Jennifer Buchanan: we started out as fellow speakers just meeting for lunch and sharing ideas, and formed this crazy, supportive, laugh-till-we-cry, mavens-got-your-back Mastermind bond that I am so grateful for. I don't know what I would do without your collective advice, support, and hilarity... not to mention (asshole alert) willingness to tolerate my (and Lisa's) occasional rants. I love you all.

Many years ago, when the idea of a next book was but a glimmer, I read a *Globe and Mail* article featuring two women who had just launched a Vancouver-based publishing company that seemed to do publishing differently... better. I vowed that if I ever wrote another book, I would seek them out because (a) their publishing concept intrigued me, (b) they're a Canadian company with international reach, and (c) they're a woman-led organization. Something about them felt right.

Fast-forward six years: with a quasi-complete manuscript and waning motivation to write, I had a conversation with Page Two Books co-founder Trena White and knew my 2013 hunch about this crew was a good one—they would help me write a better book and get it out there in a meaningful way. Thank you to everyone at Page Two who had a hand in bringing *The Success-Energy Equation* to life: Trena for bringing together the team that would work with me, and for your gentle cheerleading at every step of the process. Kendra Ward for nurturing the manuscript with your keen editor's eye and supportive writer's heart. By the time I handed over the manuscript for first-round edits I was sure I'd written a load of garbage and was so sick of looking at it that the editing process terrified me. You helped me cut, craft, and recreate until we had an end product that I'm really proud of. You're good at what you do. Thank you. And to Caela Moffet, my ever-on-top-of-it project manager; Chris Brandt, marketing strategist extraordinaire; the design team behind the cover and interior; and the eagle-eyed copy editor and proofreader: thank you for all the behind-the-scenes magic you did to bring this book to life and get it in front of readers. I'm grateful for all of you.

I can't possibly list them all, but I have a lot of great friends and supportive family that bring balance to my life and simply give me strength to do what I do with a bit more energy and focus. You all know who you are.

And to my husband, Ewan Nicholson, who nudged me along this writing process with the simple question, "How's the writing going?" and helped me work through mental blocks and low points more times than I can count. Your endless love, unconditional support, and sometimes (very) direct feedback make me better...at everything. You're my favorite.

NOTES

Introduction

1. Wan-Chen Chang and Yu-Min Ku, "The Effects of Note-Taking Skills Instruction on Elementary Students' Reading," *Journal of Educational Research* 108, no. 4 (May 2014): 1-14; Mina Rahmani and Karim Sadeghi, "Effects of Note-Taking Training on Reading Comprehension and Recall," *Reading Matrix* 11, no. 2 (April 2011), https://www.researchgate.net/publication/266074512_Effects_of_Note-Taking_Training_on_Reading_Comprehension_and_Recall.

Chapter 1

1. Carol Driver, "58% of Men Check Work Emails While on Holiday and 70% of Women Have a Problem with It (Causing a Third of Couples to Argue)," DailyMail.com, August 4, 2014, https://www.dailymail.co.uk/travel/travel_news/article-2715300/58-men-check-work-emails-holiday-70-women-problem-causing-couples-argue.html.

2. Kathryn Dill, "You're Probably Checking Your Work Email on Vacation—But You Shouldn't Be, Study Shows," *Forbes*, June 17, 2014, https://www.forbes.com/sites/kathryndill/2014/06/17/youre-probably-checking-your-work-email-on-vacation-but-you-shouldnt-be-study-shows.

3. Dan Witters and Brian Brim, "What Leaders Can Do Right Now to Optimize Worker Potential," Gallup, October 18, 2019, https://www.gallup.com/workplace/267464/leaders-right-optimize-worker-potential.aspx.

4. Jim Taylor, "Common Sense Is Neither Common nor Sense," *Psychology Today*, July 12, 2011, https://www.psychologytoday.com/ca/blog/the-power -prime/201107/common-sense-is-neither-common-nor-sense.

5. Statista, "Number of Smartphone Users Worldwide from 2016 to 2021," February 28, 2020, https://www.statista.com/statistics/330695/number -of-smartphone-users-worldwide.

6. Pew Research Center, "Mobile Fact Sheet," June 12, 2019, https://www .pewresearch.org/internet/fact-sheet/mobile; Statista, "Number of Smart- phone Users in Canada from 2013 to 2023," February 27, 2020, https://www .statista.com/statistics/467190/forecast-of-smartphone-users-in-canada.

7. *Investment Executive*, "53% of Canadians Live Paycheque to Paycheque," January 8, 2019, https://www.investmentexecutive.com/news/industry -news/53-of-canadians-live-paycheque-to-paycheque.

8. American Payroll Association, "Survey Finds Majority of Americans Live Paycheck to Paycheck," Cision PR Newswire, September 10, 2019, https:// www.prnewswire.com/news-releases/survey-finds-majority-of-americans -live-paycheck-to-paycheck-300915266.html.

Chapter 2

1. David A. Raichlen and Gene E. Alexander, "Adaptive Capacity: An Evolu- tionary Neuroscience Model Linking Exercise, Cognition, and Brain Health," *Trends in Neurosciences*, June 10, 2017, https://www.cell.com/trends/ neurosciences/fulltext/S0166-2236%2817%2930089-9; University of Arizona, "Brains Evolved to Need Exercise," *Science Daily*, June 26, 2017, https://www.sciencedaily.com/releases/2017/06/170626155729.htm.

2. National Sleep Foundation, "Sleeping at Work: Companies with Nap Rooms and Snooze-Friendly Policies," Sleep.org, https://www.sleep.org/ articles/sleeping-work-companies-nap-rooms-snooze-friendly-policies.

3. Mark R. Rosekind, Roy M. Smith, et al., "Alertness Management: Strategic Naps in Operational Settings," *Journal of Sleep Research* 4, suppl. 2 (1995): 62–66, https://onlinelibrary.wiley.com/doi/epdf/10.1111/j.1365-2869.19 95.tb00229.x.

Chapter 3

1. Mark Williamson and Renata Salecl, "Autopilot Britain," Marks and Spencer, https://corporate.marksandspencer.com/documents/reports-results -and-publications/autopilot-britain-whitepaper.pdf.

2. Courtney Seiter, "The Science of Taking Breaks at Work: How to Be More Productive by Changing the Way You Think About Downtime," Buffer, https://open.buffer.com/science-taking-breaks-at-work; *Science Daily*, "Brief Diversions Vastly Improve Focus, Researchers Find," February 8, 2011, https://www.sciencedaily.com/releases/2011/02/110208131529.htm; Kate Bartolotta, "5 Science-Backed Ways Taking a Break Boosts Our Productivity," *HuffPost*, November 16, 2016, https://www.huffpost.com/entry/5-science-backed-ways-taking-a-break-boosts-our-productivity_b_8548292.

Chapter 4

1. Paul Lewis, "'Our Minds Can Be Hijacked': The Tech Insiders Who Fear a Smartphone Dystopia," *Guardian*, October 6, 2017, https://www.theguardian.com/technology/2017/oct/05/smartphone-addiction-silicon-valley-dystopia.

2. Mike Elgan, "Smartphones Make People Distracted and Unproductive," *Computerworld*, August 12, 2017, https://www.computerworld.com/article/3215276/smartphones-make-people-distracted-and-unproductive.html; Justin Worland, "How Your Cell Phone Distracts You Even When You're Not Using It," *Time*, December 4, 2014, https://time.com/3616383/cell-phone-distraction.

3. J.S. House, K.R. Landis, and D. Umberson, "Social Relationships and Health," *Science* 241, no. 4865 (July 29, 1988): 540–45.

4. Ceylan Yeginsu, "U.K. Appoints a Minister for Loneliness," *New York Times,* January 17, 2018, https://www.nytimes.com/2018/01/17/world/europe/uk-britain-loneliness.html.

5. The Prime Minister's Office and the Office for Civil Society, "PM Commits to Government-Wide Drive to Tackle Loneliness," January 17, 2018, https://www.gov.uk/government/news/pm-commits-to-government-wide-drive-to-tackle-loneliness.

6. Eric Jaffe, "Isolating the Costs of Loneliness," Association for Psychological Science, December 1, 2008, https://www.psychologicalscience.org/observer/isolating-the-costs-of-loneliness.

7. Richard Louv, *Last Child in the Woods: Saving Our Children from Nature-Deficit Disorder* (New York: Algonquin Books, 2008).

8. Qing Li, *Forest Bathing: How Trees Can Help You Find Health and Happiness* (New York: Viking, 2018).

9.   John Medina, *Brain Rules: 12 Principles for Surviving and Thriving at Work, Home, and School* (Seattle: Pear Press, 2008).

Chapter 5

1.   Jim Collins and Jerry I. Porras, *Built to Last: Successful Habits of Visionary Companies* (New York: Harper Business, 2004).

2.   Martin Parnell, *Marathon Quest,* rev. ed. (Calgary: Rocky Mountain Books, 2018).

3.   Cyril Northcote Parkinson, "Parkinson's Law," *Economist*, November 19, 1955, https://www.economist.com/news/1955/11/19/parkinsons-law.

4.   Judith F. Bryan and Edwin A. Locke, "Parkinson's Law as a Goal-Setting Phenomenon," *Organizational Behavior and Human Performance,* August 1967, https://doi.org/10.1016/0030-5073(67)90021-9.

5.   Henry Kimsey-House, Karen Kimsey-House, Philip Sandhal, and Laura Whitworth. *Co-Active Coaching*, 4th ed. (Boston: Nicholas Brealey Publishing, 2018), 101–02.

6.   *American Heritage Dictionary of the English Language*, 5th ed., https://www.thefreedictionary.com/resonant.

Chapter 6

1.   Sarah Milne, Sheina Orbell, and Paschal Sheeran, "Combining Motivational and Volitional Interventions to Promote Exercise Participation: Protection Motivation Theory and Implementation Intentions," *British Journal of Health Psychology* 7, no. 2 (December 16, 2010), https://onlinelibrary.wiley.com/doi/abs/10.1348/135910702169420.

2.   Heidi Grant, "Get Your Team to Do What It Says It's Going to Do," *Harvard Business Review*, May 2014, https://hbr.org/2014/05/get-your-team-to-do-what-it-says-its-going-to-do.

3.   Stephen Joseph, "Unconditional Positive Regard," *Psychology Today*, October 7, 2012, https://www.psychologytoday.com/ca/blog/what-doesnt-kill-us/201210/unconditional-positive-regard.

Chapter 7

1.   Mayo Clinic, "Positive Thinking: Stop Negative Self-Talk to Reduce Stress," January 21, 2020, https://www.mayoclinic.org/healthy-lifestyle/stress-management/in-depth/positive-thinking/art-20043950.

2. Julia Scalise, "How Negative Self-Talk Sabotages Your Health and Happiness," Brain Speak, https://brainspeak.com/how-negative-self-talk-sabotages-your-health-happiness.

3. Markham Heid, "You Asked: Is It Bad for You to Read the News Constantly?" *Time*, January 31, 2018, https://time.com/5125894/is-reading-news-bad-for-you.

4. AppliedBehaviourAnalysisEdu.org, "Was Forrest Gump Autistic?" https://www.appliedbehavioranalysisedu.org/was-forrest-gump-autistic.

5. Alan Brown, "Positive Self-Talk to Feed Productivity and Tenacity," *Additude,* https://www.additudemag.com/how-to-be-your-own-life-coach-positive-self-talk; Shad Helmstetter, *What to Say When You Talk to Your Self* (New York: Gallery Books, 2017).

6. *Oxford Advanced Learner's Dictionary,* https://www.oxfordlearnersdictionaries.com/definition/english/comfort-zone.

7. Chris Desmond, "What Is Your Comfort Zone?" Medium, November 21, 2017, https://medium.com/@uncomfortableisok/what-is-your-comfort-zone-685c0bd0ed6.

8. Rick Hanson, "Stephen Colbert: We Don't Need to 'Keep Fear Alive,'" RickHanson.net, https://www.rickhanson.net/stephen-colbert-we-dont-need-to-keep-fear-alive.

9. Robert Emmons is quoted in UC Davis Health, "Gratitude is Good Medicine," UC Davis Health Medical Center, November 25, 2015, https://health.ucdavis.edu/medicalcenter/features/2015-2016/11/20151125_gratitude.html; Nils Salzgeber, "29 Scientifically Proven Benefits of Gratitude You Don't Want to Miss," NJlifehacks, June 19, 2018, https://www.njlifehacks.com/gratitude-benefits; Healthbeat, "Giving Thanks Can Make You Happier," Harvard Health Blog, https://www.health.harvard.edu/healthbeat/giving-thanks-can-make-you-happier; C. Nathan DeWall, Nathaniel M. Lambert, and Richard S. Pond Jr., "A Grateful Heart Is a Nonviolent Heart: Cross-Sectional, Experience Sampling, Longitudinal, and Experimental Evidence," *Social, Psychological, and Personality Science* 3, no. 2 (September 2011): 232–40; Nancy Digdon and Amy Koble, "Effects of Constructive Worry, Imagery Distraction, and Gratitude Interventions on Sleep Quality: A Pilot Trial," *Applied Psychology Health and Well-Being* 3, no. 2 (May 2011): 193–206.

10. Warren Berger, "The Secret Phrase Top Innovators Use," *Harvard Business Review,* September 17, 2012, https://hbr.org/2012/09/the-secret-phrase-top-innovato.

Chapter 8

1. Steven Pressfield, *Do the Work* (North Egremont, MA: Black Irish Books, 2011).

2. Kelly McGonigal, *The Willpower Instinct: How Self-Control Works, Why It Matters, and What You Can Do to Get More of It* (New York: Avery, 2011).

3. Veronika Job, Gregory M. Walton, Katharina Bernecker, and Carol S. Dweck, "Beliefs about Willpower Determine the Impact of Glucose on Self-Control," *Proceedings of the National Academy of Sciences of the United States of America,* September 10, 2013, https://www.pnas.org/content/110/37/14837.full.

4. Allan Henry, "Productivity 101: An Introduction to the Pomodoro Technique," *Lifehacker,* July 12, 2019, https://lifehacker.com/productivity-101-a-primer-to-the-pomodoro-technique-1598992730.

Chapter 9

1. Jim Loehr and Tony Schwartz, "The Making of a Corporate Athlete," *Harvard Business Review*, January 2001, https://hbr.org/2001/01/the-making-of-a-corporate-athlete.

2. Emma Seppälä, "Connect to Thrive," *Psychology Today*, August 26, 2012, https://www.psychologytoday.com/ca/blog/feeling-it/201208/connect-thrive; Emma Seppälä, *The Happiness Track: How to Apply the Science of Happiness to Accelerate Your Success* (San Francisco: HarperOne, 2016).

3. Stephanie L. Brown, Randolph M. Nesse, Amiram D. Vinokur, et al., "Providing Social Support May Be More Beneficial Than Receiving It: Results from a Prospective Study of Mortality," *Psychological Science* 14, no. 4 (July 2003): 320–27.

4. Emma Seppälä, "Connectedness and Health: The Science of Social Connection," Stanford Medicine, May 8, 2014, http://ccare.stanford.edu/uncategorized/connectedness-health-the-science-of-social-connection-infographic.

5. Jeremy Adam Smith, "Five Surprising Ways Oxytocin Shapes Your Social Life," *Greater Good Magazine*, October 17, 2013, https://greatergood.berkeley.edu/article/item/five_ways_oxytocin_might_shape_your_social_life.

6. R.F. Baumeister and M.R. Leary, "The Need to Belong: Desire for Interpersonal Attachments as a Fundamental Human Motivation," *Psychological Bulletin* 117, no. 3 (1995): 497–529.

7. National Center for Chronic Disease Prevention and Health Promotion, "Benefits of Physical Activity," Centers for Disease Control and Prevention, https://www.cdc.gov/physicalactivity/basics/pa-health/index.htm.

8. Elizabeth Anderson and Geetha Shivakumar, "Effects of Exercise and Physical Activity on Anxiety," National Center for Biotechnology Information, April 23, 2013, https://www.ncbi.nlm.nih.gov/pmc/articles/PMC 3632802.

9. Lawrence Robinson, Jeanne Segal, and Melinda Smith, "The Mental Health Benefits of Exercise," Help Guide, https://www.helpguide.org/articles/healthy-living/the-mental-health-benefits-of-exercise.htm.

10. J. Eric Ahlskog, Yonas E. Geda, Neill R. Graff-Radford, et al., "Physical Exercise as a Preventive or Disease-Modifying Treatment of Dementia and Brain Aging," National Center for Biotechnology Information, September 2011, https://www.ncbi.nlm.nih.gov/pmc/articles/PMC3258000.

11. Sama F. Sleiman, Jeffrey Henry, Rami Al-Haddad, et al., "Exercise Promotes the Expression of Brain Derived Neurotrophic Factor (BDNF) Through the Action of the Ketone Body β-Hydroxybutyrate," eLife, June 2, 2016, https://elifesciences.org/articles/15092.

12. Patrick Z. Liu and Robin Nusslock, "Exercise-Mediated Neurogenesis in the Hippocampus via BDNF," *Frontiers in Neuroscience*, February 7, 2018, https://www.frontiersin.org/articles/10.3389/fnins.2018.00052/full.

13. Wendy Suzuki and Billie Fitzpatrick, *Healthy Brain, Happy Life: A Personal Program to Activate Your Brain and Do Everything Better* (New York: HarperCollins, 2015).

14. Joyce Gomes-Osman, "What Kinds of Exercise Are Good for Brain Health?" Harvard Health Blog, May 2, 2018, https://www.health.harvard.edu/blog/what-kinds-of-exercise-are-good-for-brain-health-2018050213762.

15. Healthbeat, "A Sharper Mind: Tai Chi Can Improve Cognitive Function," Harvard Health Blog, https://www.health.harvard.edu/mind-and-mood/a-sharper-mind-tai-chi-can-improve-cognitive-function; S. Ladawan, K. Klarod, M. Philippe, et al., "Effect of Qigong Exercise on Cognitive Function, Blood Pressure, and Cardiorespiratory Fitness in Healthy Middle-Aged Subjects," *Complementary Measures in Medicine* 33 (August 2017): 39–45.

16. R. Molteni, R. Barnard, Z. Ying, C.K. Roberts, and F. Gómez-Pinilla, "A High-Fat, Refined Sugar Diet Reduces Hippocampal Brain-Derived Neurotrophic Factor, Neuronal Plasticity, and Learning," *Neuroscience* 112, no. 4 (2002): 803-14.

17. K.S. Krabbe, A.R. Nielsen, R. Krogh-Madsen, et al., "Brain-Derived Neurotrophic Factor (BDNF) and Type 2 Diabetes," *Diabetologia* 50, no. 2 (February 2007): 431-38.

18. University of Missouri, "Common Probiotics Can Reduce Stress Levels, Lessen Anxiety," November 21, 2016, https://www.sciencedaily.com/releases/2016/11/161121160038.htm; Healthbeat, "Probiotics May Help Boost Mood and Cognitive Function," Harvard Health Blog, https://www.health.harvard.edu/mind-and-mood/probiotics-may-help-boost-mood-and-cognitive-function.

19. Division of Sleep Medicine at Harvard Medical School, "Benefits of Sleep," http://healthysleep.med.harvard.edu/healthy/matters/benefits-of-sleep.

20. American Psychological Association, "More Sleep Would Make Us Happier, Healthier, and Safer," February 2014, https://www.apa.org/action/resources/research-in-action/sleep-deprivation.

21. Joshua Gowin, "Why Your Brain Needs Water," *Psychology Today*, October 15, 2010, https://www.psychologytoday.com/ca/blog/you-illuminated/201010/why-your-brain-needs-water.

22. Barry M. Popkin, Kristen E. D'Anci, and Irwin H. Rosenberg, "Water, Hydration, and Health," *Nutrition Reviews* 68, no. 8 (August 2010): 439-58; https://doi.org/10.1111/j.1753-4887.2010.00304.x.

ABOUT THE AUTHOR

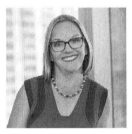

OR MORE THAN fifteen years, Michelle Cederberg has captivated audiences across North America with her empowering and humorous messages about how to set worthwhile goals and get energized for success—in business and in life.

An in-demand coach, consultant, author, and certified speaking professional, she believes that personal and professional success is directly influenced by how well we harness the physical, mental, and emotional capacity we each have within us. She helps people boost that capacity so they gain clarity, build confidence, and create the discipline to do the freakin' work.

Cederberg holds a master's in kinesiology, a BA in psychology, and a specialization in health and exercise psychology. She is a certified exercise physiologist, a certified professional Co-Active Life coach, and an ORSC-trained team coach. She truly combines mind, body, and practicality to inspire change. In addition to *The Success-Energy Equation*, she is the author of *Energy Now! Small Steps to an Energetic Life*.

Made in the USA
Middletown, DE
29 October 2020